More *Women* with ADHD
in Bite-Sized Pieces

Curbing Chaos,
Claiming Our Assets, and
Calming the Critical Self

JOAN WILDER

Copyright ©2023 by Joan Wilder

All rights reserved. This book or any portion thereof may not be reproduced or used in any manner without the express written permission of the author except for the use of brief quotations attributed to Joan Wilder in a book review or someone's website, blog, or social media account.

This book is not intended as a substitute for the medical advice of physicians. Any information on health care or health-related topics is not medical advice and should not be treated as such. The reader should regularly consult a physician or therapist in matters relating to his/her/their health and particularly with respect to the use of medications or any symptom that may require diagnosis or medical attention.

Joan Wilder
Boston, MA
joan.wilder@gmail.com

Contents

Dear Reader   9
How This Book Is   12
Thank you   14
Why Women   15
Just One More Thing   16

Part I: Trip-ups, Mismatches, and Hard Stuff   17

    What it is, Unofficially   19
    Interest-Based Motivation   23
    Distractibility   26
    Impulsivity   28
    Organizing Trouble: About Executive Functions   30
    Good Brain, Mismatched Environment   34
    Difficulty Sequencing   37
    Indecision   40
    Hyperarousal (Hyperactivity Gone Inward)   43
    Going Off on a Tangent   46
    Problems Prioritizing   48
    Emotional Dysregulation   51
    Procrastination   55
    Rejection Sensitive Dysphoria   58
    Losing Interest/Fickleness   61
    Sensory Processing Sensitivity   63
    Now and Not Now: Time Myopia   65
    Overwhelm   68
    What ADHD is, Officially   70

Part II: She What?#!: Essential ADHD Assets   73

The Orchid Hypothesis   75
Being Highly Creative and Imaginative   77
Being Highly Intuitive   80
Having the Ability to Hyperfocus   82
The Ability to Have Laser Focus Under Pressure   84
Being Improvisational, Resourceful, and Inventive   86
Having the Ability to Heal   89
Being a Catalyst   91
Being Highly Empathetic   93
Novelty-Loving   96
Being Fast Jugglers aka Multitaskers   98

Part III: The Approach/Getting Set Up   101

Take a Battle Stance   103
Celebrate Neurodiversity   104
Uncover Self Love   108
Get Diagnosed   111
Absolutely Consider Meds with an Experienced, Careful Prescriber   115
Well-Rounded Treatment Approach   118
Try a Therapist at Least a Couple Times   122
Create Structure Whenever Possible   126
Increase General Wellness   129
Find an ADHD Coach   131
Find an ADHD Buddy   135
Get Connected   136
Work on Acceptance and Allowing   140
Watch Your Hormones   143
Get Educated About ADHD   146

Connect with a Greater Good Beyond Yourself   149
Safeguard Your Feelings   151
Play   153
Grieve   156
Know that Every Little Bit Adds Up   159
Dismantle Shame   161
Strive for Simplicity   164
The Value of Failure   166
Spirit Power/Higher Flower   168
Build Your Toolbox and Leave the Rest   170

Part IV: Strategies, Tips, Hacks, and Helpful Things You Can Apply to Your Life   171

Part IV A: Organization, Planning, and Memory   173

Landing Pad   175
Use External Cues   176
Desk Notebook (Info Capture System)   178
Notes App (on Apple Devices)   181
Brain Dump (Clearing Your Cache and Resetting Your Cookies)   183
Pros and Cons List   186
Your Own Digital Filing Cabinet   187
Computer Bookmarks and Favorites Bars   188
Out of Sight, Out of Mind   191
Cleaning, Server-Style   192
Daily To-Do List (Staying Present to the Day's Needs)   194
A Way to Save Passwords   196
One Credit Card   197
Gift-Giving Hack   198
F*ck it   200

Part IV B: Time Management — 201

Prepping Things — 203
Prioritizing What's Important — 206
Chunking — 209
Transitioning — 212
Analog Clocks — 215
Big Whiteboard — 216
Jot Everything Down — 218
Scheduling — 219
My Beloved Timer Tool — 221

Part IV C: Self-Knowledge — 223

Self-Inventory — 225
Talking Nice About All Our Brains — 228
Excavate Your Authentic Self, Part 1: How We May Have Lost Ourselves — 230
Excavate Your Authentic Self, Part 2: What You Like, What You Don't Like, and More — 233
Dwell on the Good — 236
Let Go of Perfection — 238
Allow Grace — 240
Develop Your Observer — 242
Tiny Gratitude List — 244
Use a Journal — 245
Consider a Digital Journal (If You Change Your Mind About a Paper One) — 248
Best Environments for You — 250

Part IV D: Self Care — 253

Not So Hard! (What Stress is and Does to Us) — 255

One Push Up	258
Forest Bathing	260
Use Your Subconscious	262
Affirmations/Self Talk	264
Groundhog Day with a Difference	267
Create Slogans	269
Seasonal Affective Disorder Lamps (Let the Light Shine)	270
Control Screen Time	272
One Formula for Making a Change	274
Frozen Vegetables: Seriously	276
Get Dressed First Thing in the Morning	277
Make Your Bed	279
Sit on the Floor for a Minute	280
Consider Yoga	282
Fidgeting Can Help	286
Exercise for Short Bursts Throughout the Day	287
Be Your Own Friend	289
Begin Again	291
Tiny Sensory Sensitivity Hack When Shopping	293
Suiting Up and Showing Up	294
God Box	296

Part IV E: Feelings — **299**

Breaking Through Discouragement—and Addiction	301
About Anxiety	303
Breathing	305
Dealing with Anger	306
Courage	308
Forgiveness	309
One Way to Get Around Emotional Dysregulation: Do You Want to be Happy, or Right?	312

Off Days: Out Sick with ADHD (Take a Mental Health Day)   314
Bathrooms as Sanctuaries   316

Part IV F: Relationships   **319**

The Pause Button   321
About Apologizing   324
The Desire to Hit Send   326
Stop People Pleasing   327
Asking for Help   329
Body Doubling   331
Bookending   334
Use a Therapist as an ADHD Coach   335
Find Your Tribe   336
Ask for a Moment to Shift Gears   339
Take Notes   341
Help With Interrupting   342
Take the Best, Leave the Rest   344
One Last Thing   345

Resources   *347*
An Informal Index   *357*
About the Author   *363*

Dear Reader

It's been six years since I wrote my tiny book, *Help for Women with ADHD: My Simple Strategies for Conquering Chaos*, and some things haven't changed!

For instance: I just popped into the bathroom, pulled down my pants to pee, then instead, grabbed the laundry basket—real quick—and loaded the washing machine, bare-assed!, my jeans hanging around my knees.

Yes: I still do things like that, but overall my life has improved a lot as a result of the continuing awareness that I have ADHD. Two things stand out as the biggest treasures I've uncovered.

One is a **strong commitment to working on loving myself and all neurodivergent people** regardless of our invisible differences.

It's a rich world with all kinds of people and brains, yet our dominant culture has denigrated differences and catered to a narrow, conventional set of standards that dismisses ADHDers as outsiders who don't fit in.

But the ADHD brain isn't a mistake, it's an expression of the diversity in nature that makes all living systems healthy and resilient. Some experts believe that the high-spirited ADHD brain has always been around and is largely responsible for seeding humankind with sparks of creativity, invention, and discovery.

Which isn't to say that ADHD doesn't challenge us, it absolutely does. But it's important to recognize that many of these challenges arise from living in a culture that hasn't learned to interpret our **stylistic differences!**

Meanwhile, though, the other great thing I've realized is that the **positive traits** that almost always come with ADHD are substantial and important. They're not just little inconsequential talents people mention to make ADHDers feel better.

No: They're big energies, traits, and ways of being.

Interestingly, the assets that come with ADHD are pretty much the flip side of the same energies and traits that challenge us—and are too often buried beneath them.

For instance, the same wide, **unfiltered focus** that is so distracting for ADHDers also fuels the ability to **improvise and innovate.** The same **love of novelty** that leaves you with a mountain of commitments can also have you **walking into a new discovery.** And, the **disorganization** that keeps you scrambling after items you've lost is the same energy as the **creative chaos** that leads to producing **imaginative new creations.**

I'm not saying we're all geniuses, but I am saying that ADHDers have something very special.

All of which is to say that everything we can do to accept and love ourselves just as we are—while also supporting ourselves however we can—will help our assets blossom.

I hope that knowing we're vessels for important energies also helps you dismantle the low self-esteem that often accompanies a lifetime of not fitting into society's conventional norms.

So, wherever you are and whatever you're doing—whether you're in good shape or struggling—my biggest wish is that you know that **we are all—absolutely, bottom line, no-matter-what—totally deserving human beings like everybody else**, whether we've forgotten some project, didn't get the house together, talked the entire time, blew the money, missed the interview, or never showed up at all!

How This Book Is

I can't stand prefaces and forwards in books. I like to get right into the nitty-gritty but there are a couple things I have to explain!

This book has 140 entries (short chapters). Each one stands alone.

By that, I mean that **you can open the book at random and read any single piece. If one doesn't appeal to you, you can try another.** (Or you could read the whole book, front to back, which would be even better!)

Most of all, I want the book to be like a safe friend you can turn to when you need a little help remembering that you're not alone.

The entries range from one to four pages long.

I've roughly grouped them into the four parts below.

Part I: Trip-ups, Mismatches, and Difficulties

Each of these entries is about how the challenging parts of ADHD sometimes feel. The idea here is that by describing and sharing my challenging ADHD traits, you'll see yourself in some of them. Connecting with others in the same boat works magic for me. I hope it does for you, too.

Part II: She What?!#: Essential ADHD Assets

Each of the entries here is about one of ADHD's assets—as I see them. My hope is that by teasing them apart and identifying them individually, you'll come to recognize the powerful energies within yourself and be inspired to call them forth! Not only that, but being aware of your assets may motivate you to get support harnessing your challenges so your assets can flower!

Part III: The Approach: Getting Set Up

The 24 entries here are about positioning yourself—physically, emotionally, psychologically, and spiritually—toward ADHD and the fact of your having ADHD. They also offer ways to situate yourself in various environments so you feel supported in a world that can hold you and your ADHD in a loving way.

Part IV: Strategies, Tips, Hacks, and Helpful Things You Can Apply to Your Life

The entries here contain tips, tools, strategies, and suggestions that help me manage the whirling chaos of the world.

They're lightly subdivided into "Organization," "Time Management," "Self Knowledge," "Self-care," "Feelings," and "Relationships."

If you open the book at random and don't see a bold title, flip backwards or forwards to find an entry's first page.

Thanks for being here: I think about you all the time.

Thank you

My deepest thanks to all the women whose stories and anecdotes are scattered around this book in italics!

I've culled these little "shares" from emails, phone calls, and Zooms I've had with women who wrote to me about my first book and other women with ADHD I've encountered here and there.

Each woman is identified by her first name and sometimes a bit more personal info, as per her wishes.

Why Women

I wrote this book for and about women with ADHD not because I wish to exclude men, but because I relate to women with ADHD. I know women with ADHD. I feel safe and at home with women with ADHD. *I love women with ADHD.*

Just One More Thing

I'm in no way an expert on ADHD! I'm just writing here about what ADHD feels like to me, what I think about it, what I've learned, and how I experience its effects.

Look—before you go any further, remember this: Nobody—not even the best expert—can tell you that your ADHD makes you this, that, or the other thing!

Minds are mostly a mystery—brains too—and science can never account for the wisdom in a woman's heart.

We're so much more than any ADHD label!

Each of us is an intricate tapestry and the strands of ADHD that run through us are only one type of thread among the millions that comprise the unique pattern that is you.

The most important thing to know is that you're a child of this world with *a heart that can love, just like everybody else.*

All the rest is nothing next to the treasure that is your heart. *Don't forget.*

PART I

Trip-ups, Mismatches, and Hard Stuff

Each of these entries is about how the challenging parts of ADHD sometimes feel. The idea here is that by describing and sharing my challenging ADHD traits, you'll see yourself in some of them and feel less alone. Connecting with others who are in the same boat works magic for me. I hope it does for you, too.

What it is, Unofficially

A kid in a toy store.

Can you imagine the scene? Her little eyes are wide as she takes in thousands of dolls, games, books, bikes, skates, and a million more toys: Everything a jumble of color, shape, sound and oh! dollhouses with hundreds of miniature things to go in them!

This is close to the kind of head I wake up to every day.

Contrary to what the name Attention Deficit Hyperactivity Disorder (ADHD) implies, the majority of us do not have a deficit of attention. In fact, **the ADHD mind pays too much attention to too many things at once.** It has a wide-open focus, registering large swaths of input from wherever we are. And, without the filters that allow neurotypical people to blur out the background stuff, our bright minds swim in a rich distracting sea of all types of awareness.

The name ADHD is also misleading because not all women with ADHD are hyperactive. And, in the majority of us who are, the hyperactivity almost always operates internally, creating what's called hyperarousal.

All of which can leave some women with ADHD adrift, unable to keep their heads above water, lost to action in a world of dreamy thoughts. Others are tossed here and there internally, their interest grabbed by one thing after another: (Which is why

I end up doing things like loading the washing machine with my jeans around my knees when I've gone into the bathroom just to pee.)

Without awareness or support, the ADHD brain can generate a range of challenging behaviors that make it hard to manage your time, make plans, get started on a task, follow through, organize your belongings, or remember what you promised you'd do.

Experts generally sum up ADHD as a neurobiological condition that stems from uncommon levels of distractibility, impulsivity, and hyperactivity.

ADHD is also known as a spectrum disorder because not everyone with it displays all the characteristic behaviors that are used to define it. ADHD comprises a large umbrella of traits, and some of us have some of the traits while others of us have different ones.

Not only that, it's also important to understand that all people experience the same traits that women with ADHD have, but to a lesser extent. Part of getting diagnosed involves ascertaining how strongly and for how long a person experiences the many characteristics that define the disorder.

ADHD women are sensitive perceivers and responders, and our genetic makeup gives us an enhanced response to our environments—good and bad.

Too often, unless we are lucky enough to have enlightened teachers or parents who recognize the value of diversity in brains, we are shamed for our differences. Now, at the dawn of the neurodivergent movement, our differences can be recognized, invited in, and contribute their unique perspectives to the world.

When acknowledged and seen, women with ADHD can flower brilliantly.

Yup, the same characteristic ADHD energies that challenge us can also generate constructive abilities, or assets. **I can sometimes spot a woman with ADHD just as easily by her assets—** her big imagination, creativity, strong intuition, ingenuity, adventurousness, curiosity—as her challenges.

There's no single, conclusive test that proves you have ADHD. Diagnoses are made by a mental health professional (psychiatrist, psychologist, neurologist, clinical social worker, or therapist) taking a detailed evaluation.

Still, you can get an idea of where you stand by taking a look at the classic characteristics you experience with regularity.

A quick look at the most characteristic traits of women with ADHD:

- Difficulty prioritizing, deciding, and choosing, which results in a general feeling of being overwhelmed.
- Highly aware of their surroundings; imaginative and creative.
- Easily distracted from a task at hand.
- Passionate and enthusiastic for the new and the unknown.
- Difficulty getting motivated to start on a chosen task.
- Tendency to misplace things often and feel disorganized.
- Ability to see outside the box and be innovative.
- Having oversized emotional responses.

- Able to focus hard, work fast, and accomplish a lot, especially when they love what they're doing.
- Losing time: slipping into an alternate time zone, running late, feeling rushed.
- Empathetic, enthusiastic, optimistic, and big-hearted.
- Difficulty taking a step-by-step approach to a problem.
- Ability to see the whole picture: highly intuitive.

Can you relate?

Interest-Based Motivation

In the course of a single day, I can move mountains on something I'm interested in, yet be unable to lift a finger to start on something that doesn't interest me—even if that thing is important.

Many prominent ADHD experts believe that one of the most-defining characteristics of the ADHD nervous system is that it is interest-based.

This means that an ADHDer is motivated by what interests her and not by the importance of a task.

In contrast, those with **neurotypical** (normal/most common) brains are able to become sufficiently motivated to take action, even when they have no interest in a task. For them, it's motivating enough to know that a particular task is important and that there will be consequences—good (tax money refunded, kudos from co-workers, pleasing your mate) if they do it, or bad (loss of a job, breaking a promise, being late) if they don't do it.

But concepts of obligation, duty, importance and even negative consequences are often not enough to motivate the ADHD brain to act on boring or routine tasks.

Instead, the ADHD brain is largely stimulated by what's new, competitive, exciting, creative, challenging, or urgent. The great part of this ADHD interest-based brain is that it can really go to town when it's motivated, often surging into states of hyperfocus that allows it to delve deeply into an issue where it can mine rare insights, ideas, and the fruits of high productivity.

Still, **finding ways to get motivated is essential for ADHDers,** and it goes without saying that a lot of the strategies in any good ADHD treatment plan involve motivation.

I always marvel at how my neurotypical sister-in-law, Ande, and my friend Jane, for instance, just do what they have to do without a big struggle. This allows them to keep up with all of life's BS without expending a massive amount of energy.

Not me. I can go weeks without even getting close to thinking about that thing that needs doing way in the back—of the back—of my mind. The Department of Motor Vehicles sent me a form about renewing my driver's license last year that sat on my desk unread for months after my license had expired. *I knew it was there, but I couldn't. I didn't want to, I couldn't. Then, after having avoided it for a while, the idea to do it moved into another deeper place in my mind that felt very far away and lost.*

So often ADHDers are accused of being lazy, but it isn't that!

Various experiments have shown that brains are stimulated into a motivated state when they are adequately supplied by the release of different **brain chemicals**, known as **neurotransmitters, especially dopamine and norepinephrine.**

So, when the ADHD brain is unable to get motivated, it's partly because it is not releasing enough dopamine to excite/stimulate the brain to take action!

The average Joe, on the other hand, is able to deploy their attention sufficiently to accomplish uninteresting chores *because their brain has adequate supplies of neurotransmitters.*

Learning which environments stimulate me and putting myself in those environments is one of the many strategies I use to get myself stimulated enough to tackle all the tasks I need to do.

A lot of other strategies for tackling a lack of stimulation are sprinkled through this book, especially in Part IV.

Distractibility

> *"To me, everything is interesting,"* said Mandy, a former school administrator with ADHD. *"My mind and thoughts race fast. They are hard to control and I cannot help but share them because ... they feel so exciting, like I've discovered or uncovered something. So, if it's when we are supposed to be focusing on this one area that we have this explosion of thoughts that are related to this intended area of focus, why not dive in and explore these areas? **This is what it feels like to me—like I'm an explorer being told not to do any exploring.**"*
>
> —Mandy, self-employed, mother of two daughters

It helps to see how distracted we can become from a task at hand when you understand that the ADHD mind roams far and wide, taking in everything, and gushing with ideas. **This hyper-awareness of the environment is one of the hallmark characteristics of people with ADHD and one of the main roots of distraction.**

Some Internet memes say that ADHD is like living in a mind that has several radio stations on at once. The great ADHD pioneer, psychiatrist, and warm-hearted ADHDer Edward Hallowell, M.D., maintains that ADHD is like having a race car brain and poor brakes. And I've always felt it's like being a great orchestra with a weak conductor.

So, it's no wonder things grab hold of your head out of nowhere and snag your attention. It happens to me all the time. I'll be a few sentences into a conversation with a friend and suddenly interject how gorgeous the color of her scarf is, that she won't believe what I made for dinner, or that tomorrow is forecast to be sunny!

Distractions from your environment can grab your attention—loud noises, competing conversations, movement, a messy desk—or from within your head: daydreams, desires, impulses, and more.

Naturally, with such a wide awareness, it can be hard to stay focused on one particular thing! In contrast, the neurotypical mind has fewer things vying for its attention. All of which lowers the distraction factor for them.

Being overly stimulated by all you see, hear, feel, and think makes it hard to focus on one thing.

It's encouraging to understand that everything you do to manage your difficult ADHD traits will add up and help you channel the powerful energy behind your distractibility in constructive ways.

Impulsivity

I did something impulsive one recent early evening. I didn't even see it coming until the words were out of my mouth!

Bubbling over with an excited sense of connection and happiness from having had a good talk with my neighbors earlier in the day (it's May 4, 2020, and we're quarantining), I yelled out the window that I'd found out that a favorite restaurant was doing takeout and that I was going to buy them dinner.

Impulsivity is acting before you think. Some people call it being spontaneous or uninhibited. True, but it can get you in a lot of fixes you don't want to be in.

Overwhelming impulses partner with other common ADHD traits, including the tendency to have big, emotion-packed, adrenalin pumping responses to events and situations—commonly referred to as hyperarousal. I can get so inwardly hyperactive with excitement about something that I'm bursting. This excitement demands an immediate release, like the satisfaction of blurting something out, hitting the "send" key, or doing something sudden and unexpected.

If I don't have any strategies in place for reining in my excited impulses, they can cause me to fly all over the place. I'll want to do or check out this, that, or the other thing, and abandon whatever I'm doing to follow some impulse somewhere. **This results

in a pattern of chronic starting and stopping as I fly off to respond to a new idea or desire and then quit that one, too, to fly off to another.

So much starting and stopping creates a whole lot of unfinished stuff in your head that can make you feel very overwhelmed.

So, what happened with the neighbors? After having yelled out my intention to bring them dinner, I realized I had a whole dinner already planned—chicken defrosted, broccoli already sautéed, lettuce that needed eating. And I hadn't said *when* I was going to bring them dinner. So, I figured I'd do it another time. But, soon after that, the neighbor-wife's sister died unexpectedly, and I knew she was grieving. So that didn't seem like the right time to drop off some celebratory takeout. And then, and then. And then….

I never did it. I just never did it.

All I can really do now is hope they think they must have misheard me!

Organizing Trouble: About Executive Functions

"Even with medication, ADHD had an impact on my schoolwork. Becoming aware of how I best learn was very helpful. I have found that for me to fully understand the material, I would need to hear it, then repeat it in my own words to make sure I heard the information correctly and comprehended what I was learning.

In graduate school, I recorded my lectures and would listen to them, stop them as needed in order to write down my notes (neatly) and understand the material. Listening to a 60-minute lecture would take me 90 minutes or more to get through. But again, although time consuming, it was what I felt I needed to do to in order to receive, understand, and retain the information."

—Julie, physical therapist in the UK

Many experts say that most ADHDers have higher-than-average intelligence.

Meanwhile, though, quite apart from our intelligence, is a group of helper abilities just beneath our conscious awareness. These abilities act like little computer widgets, functioning automatically behind the scenes to facilitate how we organize and undertake everything we do.

In psychology, these operations are called executive functions.

These nearly automatic functions include what's called working memory, which is the ability to hold many thoughts in mind around a particular task over time. Also operating in the realm of executive functions are underlying sorting, organizing, and prioritizing abilities. These allow us to easily deconstruct tasks into the steps we need to take to identify, approach, and initiate the actions required to accomplish specific goals. (Breaking down tasks into steps is often referred to as chunking or sequencing.)

Also included among the executive functions are the self-awareness to track your progress, sustain action toward a task at hand, and the ability to regulate strong emotions, like frustration, so as to maintain focus.

Some experts find it useful to think of ADHD as a condition that causes deficits in one or more of our executive functions.

Again, it's not a deficit in our intelligence, it's a deficit in the internal cues that allow us to accomplish what we want to do.

Don't get scared: This is nothing new to us. It's just an alternate way of understanding what's already so familiar: that we often have difficulty starting on tasks we have no interest in, prioritizing what's important, organizing what steps to take next, forgetting things, and following through.

The great value in knowing about executive functioning in ADHDers is that it illustrates **how useful it is for us to employ external cues in our environment** to compensate for deficits in these internal cues.

Like **Post-Its**! And **whiteboards**! Lots of **analog clocks** and **alarms**! **Lists** of goals, posted where you can see them. **Words written on mirrors** or taped to the inside of a closet door or another private place. **Images of a final product** or goal completed. The creation of **mind maps**, or **picture collages** of what you're working on. Creating and checking in often with your **daily journal**, **planner**, notebook, computer app, or wherever you store information.

Executive functions come into play with everything from packing lunch to designing a rocket ship.

It's no wonder that lots of women with ADHD don't get diagnosed until they become mothers, a role that demands so much executive functioning that it tips them over the brink.

Just picking up kids from school relies on a range of these inner cues that enable us to visualize and hold in our minds all that's required to get the job done.

To do anything, we need to be able to sort, plan, and initiate many awarenesses and tasks. In the above example, it might include remembering that one kid is getting out late because of soccer practice; that the school has new procedures for car pickups; that we have to get the time off to do the pick-up. We also need to know where the car keys are; make and take the needed snacks or soccer equipment; be aware whether we have food in the house for said snacks; carve out time to prepare said food; be appropriately dressed; have money or the required paperwork we might need and have completed said paperwork.

All these things can be sorted so helpfully using external cues.

The biggest takeaway here, for me, is to never underestimate how useful external cues are!

Good Brain, Mismatched Environment

"Everybody is a genius. But if you judge a fish by its ability to climb a tree, it will live its whole life believing that it is stupid."

—Unknown

"She is that smart kid that thinks she's stupid. They tell her she's lazy and would be successful if she would only try. They might as well tell her to spread her arms and fly.

When she finally breaks free of their mold, they can't believe what she really is. Like the butterfly surprising the caterpillar, she is so much more: If only they'd just let her be herself."

—Bethenie, entrepreneur

Our dominant (Western) society functions in a linear, one-thing-after-another way.

This means society approaches and organizes tasks by how important they are and what needs to be done first.

At work, in social settings, at parent meetings, conferences, on the phone—we're expected to tackle things in a culturally agreed upon, orderly manner.

We're expected to wait our turn, stay on topic, be amiable, composed, and cheerful—*but not too cheerful***—and act at a certain pace: neither too slowly nor too quickly.**

It's second nature for neurotypical women to break down tasks into a series of steps, and approach problems and issues in an ordered manner.

ADHD women, on the other hand, are more likely to (intuit and) grasp the big picture surrounding an issue and jump right into it and start working away at many parts of it all at once.

This tendency—to tackle issues from a **wholistic point of view**—makes it hard for women with ADHD to fit into a culture where orderly, measured execution is the expected approach.

This makes syncing with the world—a job, family, relationships, community—difficult and often fraught with failure or misunderstanding.

In childhood, unless you're blessed with aware parents or teachers, **you end up having your assets buried while you struggle to be understood and fit in.**

Several ADHD traits tend ADHDers to behave in other eccentric (not common/uncommon) ways (compared with society's expected behavior patterns).

For instance, we can appear to be off the beam in a meeting when we come up with some aspect of a problem that others

35

haven't yet foreseen. We can also feel so impassioned about our ideas that we interject them with a heightened excitement that feels chaotic and confounding to people habituated to taking an organized, rational, step-by-step approach.

It's a difference in style.

You know how enlightened educators offer students lessons that are tailored to their different learning styles (auditory, visual, kinetic)? Well, it's like that: **Society can come to support and cultivate the value in ADHD brains by accommodating them in various ways.**

Luckily, the neurodiversity movement is helping communities realize that they benefit from the different points of view and talents inherent in ADHD (and other types of) brains. It's also expanding the ways we recognize intelligence itself.

Where and when we give ADHDers the freedom to work differently—and society learns that solutions can arise in offbeat rhythms—ADHDers will be able to more fully, rightfully enrich our communities.

Difficulty Sequencing

I'd been wanting to make a small, raised garden bed for several weeks when I got up the other day.

As usual, I wasn't sure where to start: The whole project was a jumble to me.

Breaking down a task into the action steps you need to take to accomplish it is called sequencing. I have trouble with it.

Meanwhile, though, I really wanted to make this raised bed!

So… I corralled all the patience I could and wrote down a list of things I could think of that I'd need: a construction plan for sure; wood cut to size from the lumber yard; screws or brackets to hold the corners together; a place to put the bed and what tools I'd need to dig up the grass to prep the site; what kind of compost or manure I'd need to enrich the soil and how much I'd need. All this and more.

And it was raining. And I couldn't get the garden built all in one day (my preferred modus operandi) which was a real turnoff to my brain.

But because I'd broken down the task into the steps I'd need to take, I f*cking saw, from my list, that one thing I could do right then was decide how I was going to build it.

So I went online and found an easy plan for a rectangular 4-foot by 8-foot frame, screwed together with 3-inch "deck screws" and decided to do it that way.

Then, I copied down the wood sizes and deck-screw size I'd need (in the notebook I always have with me).

And even though I felt at loose ends about the whole thing, I went to the lumber yard and bought the screws and had the wood cut into the lengths I'd need. (Our lumber yard has a great shop and they'll cut wood for you.)

It felt unfulfilling, but the next day, when I woke up, I HAD THE WOOD and a big head start to getting the thing made! And I made it—thanks to my step by step approach!

When I said, above, that I have a problem sequencing, I have to remember that, in fact, my sequencing ability is operating all the time and that my challenges with sequencing arise when doing something unfamiliar.

I mean, dozens of nearly unconscious thoughts and connections occur inside our heads as we take action on everything we do all the time.

Even just getting up and walking outside, say: You have to push up off the chair, stand up, head in the right direction, take a step, continue walking, grab the door handle, step over the landing, and close the door behind you. It's second nature for our brains to break down each of these actions into the multiple steps each comprises!

So, the ADHD brain is able to sequence well every day as we move through the habitual basics of our lives, but it can have

real difficulty sequencing the steps required for unfamiliar and new tasks.

Just recognizing this is half the battle.

Indecision

"Too many options FREAK me out. My mind fights itself. I only wanted a loaf of bread!"

—Selina Danielle, UK

"Making a decision has always been a struggle with me. It has even been extremely emotional and debilitating where I just lay on my bed and cry because I cannot make a decision. When it gets to that point, I typically reach out to someone to talk it out and discuss the pros and cons of each choice. A lot of times, I've had difficulty deciding what to do or choosing to attend one event over another, but it can also be something like what to eat for dinner. What has helped me with this is being honest with myself. Typically, I WANT to do something but feel obligated to do the other. Now I try to make the decision based on what I really want and have realized that whatever I choose I need to accept and not dwell on the other option."

—Julie

I'd say that **being indecisive is one of my hardest traits**. Often, I just simply cannot choose among options.

Listen to this story: I'll make it short even though it played out in time for at least eight weeks.

Over the winter holidays this year (2022), I had to buy a new computer, and I could not decide among many different models. And what happened, believe it or not, is that **I actually ended up buying and returning five different MacBooks before settling on the sixth and final choice.** I mean I paid for each one, took it home and laboriously set it up with all my apps and passwords. Then, deciding I didn't want it, I painstakingly erased everything back to the thing's factory settings, reboxed it carefully, and went to the store to return it. I was unsure about each one for different reasons: One was too heavy, one's screen was too small, one didn't have the newest processor, one was so expensive I thought I better not spend all that money. I wasn't even sure which color to get!

And the whole ordeal was prolonged because the return policy for everything was extended way beyond the normal two weeks for the holidays. I was in an agony of (first-world) indecision: I could not decide which one to keep. I spread my purchases between Best Buy and the Apple store and managed to not embarrass myself as much as you would think returning them all. (The people in the stores don't actually care.)

I did everything I knew to do: wrote lots of pros and cons lists on these computers and learned all the specs of each so that I was correcting sales people about their weight and size. I'd ask random people in the stores which one they'd choose, hoping to get a message from the Universe. Nothing helped. I kept thinking I'd be better off with the bigger one, the smaller one, the big one but with the older chip, the silver one, the gray one.

My godchild Lily helped. She said that whichever computer I decided on wouldn't be perfect and that they were all great.

So, trying to snap myself out of this ridiculousness, I started affirming that all the computers were phenomenal machines and I loved them all. And I finally decided—and thank God the post-holiday return policy finally expired—and the whole thing was over.

My indecision in this case was because I was afraid of making a mistake on something so expensive—and having to live regretting my choice.

Other times, we can't make a decision because we're worried about what other people will think of our choice. Or we have too much on our plates and feel overwhelmed.

Another big block to deciding is that **I always want to do everything first—right now—which jams me up.** This is part of the ADHD trait of time myopia or time blindness.

Another thing that skews my ability to prioritize what I want most when making decisions is **my love of going after something new**. I'll put extra weight on some choice because it's new, even though, in the back of my head, I know it's not the most important thing for me to do or choose to do, so that messes with my ability to decide.

Sometimes I can't decide because **I'm afraid of missing out on something**. Or that I won't be able to accomplish my choice. Or I'm worried about the finances of the thing: Can I afford it?

But whatever the reasons, it feels like I just can't decide!

Hyperarousal (Hyperactivity Gone Inward)

Even though I was criticized as a kid for being "speedy," most of that external hyperactivity is now internal. Every morning, pretty much, I'm all revved up and ready to go!

My mind gushes with urges to do so many things, big and small, long term and short—a million desires.

Sound familiar? It's a restlessness that wants to do everything.

This internal hyperactivity is known as hyperarousal. It causes me to think long and hard about too much, feel strongly about even insignificant things, and be bursting with an enthusiasm and need to express myself.

All of which sometimes jams me up from starting on any single thing.

It feels as though hyperarousal underlies almost all the core ADHD traits I experience.

For one, it fuels my hyper-vigilant way of taking in the world—how I'm always "open for business" interacting with my environment in my head: that strong attraction I have to leap for and mentally grab hold of every little passing distraction that comes to mind.

Hyperarousal definitely fuels my impulsivity—those times I can't contain my desire to do or say something.

It's also behind my difficulty managing my strong emotional responses to so much of what happens in any day: Good and bad.

Many women with ADHD are very sensitive perceivers, registering almost everything with a high intensity.

All this has me, often, responding to a friend or others intensely: loudly, enthusiastically, emotionally, quickly, irritably, impulsively, and with strong words.

Even though I'm aware that I do this, I get caught up doing it anyway. A very close friend, every once in a while, will tell me to lower my voice. (I always appreciate her reminder.)

I get very excited around people I love and want to tell them everything.

One time, after 10 minutes on the phone trying to organize help for a mutual friend in a remote hospital, this acquaintance-guy stopped the whole conversation and told me that I sounded so angry.

But I wasn't angry at all, I was just excited about what we were planning.

After he said that, I bent over backwards to tell him (effortfully keeping my voice low and my pace slow) what I was like: that I can come across sometimes like I'm angry when all I am is wildly impassioned! And that I was sorry. And that I wasn't mad at him in the least little bit. But that I get excited. And forceful.

All energies can be channeled for the good or bad, so I appreciate that hyperarousal is also responsible for so much good: spontaneity, creativity, an adventurous spirit that forges ahead into new territory, and more.

Again, hyperarousal has to do with having a fast brain and difficulty inhibiting all the thoughts and emotions it generates. Learn to recognize it.

Going Off on a Tangent

I loved **this great cartoon** someone posted on Instagram.

It was a picture of **P. Diddy in a sound studio seated at a massive music control board** with hundreds of colorful buttons and levers. He had on earphones.

And the caption was, *"Me making a playlist for a five-minute shower."*

This is a **hilarious** example of the ADHD trait of getting distracted by something—and then becoming so deeply absorbed by the new interest that we don't want to stop: that it sort of hurts to stop.

This cartoon exemplifies how our attentional abilities lack fluidity: It can be both difficult for us to deploy our attention and then difficult to withdraw it.

ADHDers have eclectic and wide-ranging interests and a magnetic attraction to them.

Once I start exploring something, it's hard to pull myself back.

The trick for me most of the time is to "rip off the band-aid," if I possibly can.

In other words, if I become aware that I'm off on a tangent I abruptly stop what I'm doing and immediately jump into something else to break the attraction (to the object of my deep dive)—like jumping around, putting on some music, getting a glass of water, checking my to-do list.

Generally, once I do that, I can get into the next thing.

Problems Prioritizing

Similar to my chronic indecision, I've spent much of my life without ever consciously prioritizing what I wanted or needed the most. As Jim, my old therapist, observed, I used to respond to everything with equal weight: dust balls, a cousin's newborn, asteroids, sour milk.

I now see that I moved through life by intuiting what my next move should be. And, thank God, my intuition is good. But, it wasn't the most effective way to get where I wanted to go.

Many women with ADHD, like me, have difficulty identifying the difference in importance among all the things they might do in a single day.

This disinclination to discriminate between what matters and what doesn't leaves us susceptible to squandering all our energy on whatever grabs our attention.

And, what generally grabs my attention, on a given day, is something that feels, or actually is, urgent. Like dropping off your kid's lunch real quick; writing a report for your boss you've put off; following an irresistible impulse to join the gym and start weight training.

The high energy of doing things urgently can make you feel like you're really accomplishing something—and sometimes you are. Life requires us to do all kinds of things everyday. But plenty of times an urgent task doesn't matter at all and accomplishes nothing!

The little secret to building a life you want (a little bit at a time) is the fact that **not everything that appears to be urgent is important!**

This is a big issue with the time management pundits and I find it so useful. They advise that we ask ourselves three questions of any task that faces us:

- Is it urgent and important?
- Is it urgent and not important?
- *Is it not urgent but very important?*

If the thing is urgent *and* important, then you need to get it done. But, if the thing is urgent *and not important*, you can cross that f*cker off your list!

And, finally, *if the thing is urgent and very important*, then you've found something you can do that day that will build on your lifetime goals and dreams.

To do this, though, you have to have dug deeply and identified your overall lifetime priorities.

These are the things that give your life meaning: ways of being you strive to embody over time. Being kind, forgiving, loving. Raising a family. Taking soup to your sick neighbor. Working for a cause. The list is endless.

The useful thing about identifying these big lifetime priorities is that once you have, they help you cut right through to the truth when prioritizing among things to do on any given day.

I love that identifying your overarching lifetime priorities—what you want to build over time—gives both purpose to your life and direction to your days.

Very helpful!

Emotional Dysregulation

My friend—I'll call her Emma—looks to all the world like a together, pretty, younger woman. And she is all those things, and she's also a person who—like me—**sometimes gets painfully overwhelmed by supersized, negative emotions that come on seemingly out of nowhere.**

I don't know what the statistics are on how many women with ADHD struggle with what's called emotional dysregulation, but I know that I have and do.

What it is, is the eruption of strong negative emotion that comes on quickly: You can become totally flooded with anger, resentment, jealousy, rejection, or some other painful emotion, in a flash. It's the emotional equivalent of getting hit by a truck out of nowhere or going from zero to sixty in a second.

It's so important to recognize that emotional dysregulation is often part of ADHD because you don't hear much about it, yet many of us have it. In fact, girls with ADHD often get misdiagnosed as bipolar by therapists who don't recognize that their struggles to regulate their strong emotions stem from their ADHD nervous systems.

Other people with various neurodiversities also suffer with this difficulty regulating the overwhelming emotions their brains perceive.

My understanding of the **science** behind emotional dysregulation is very limited. I've read that it arises because the **part of the brain that registers emotions (amygdala) can be overactive, and the part that regulates and inhibits emotions (frontal cortex) can be underactive.**

I've also read that **emotional dysregulation can result from problems between the brain's cerebellum and the inner ear.** These two parts of our heads work together to form the **vestibulocerebellar system, or VCS**, which has long been known to be responsible for our ability to keep our physical balance.

Now, research cited in *ADHD 2.0*, by Edward M. Hallowell, M.D., and John J. Ratey, M.D., **finds the VCS responsible not only for regulating our physical balance, but for regulating our emotional balance, as well!** The authors recommend various (physical) **balancing exercises** as a way to improve emotional balance and other ADHD symptoms. (Please see Chapter 3 in the above-mentioned book for more on how the cerebellum appears to be responsible for many ADHD symptoms, not only emotional dysregulation.)

All of which is to say what some of us already know: **We have a reactive hypersensitivity to life coupled with underactive self-regulation that can produce strong negative emotions that bury us, taking center stage over everything else.** It's a painful, sometimes debilitating, state of being.

If I don't attend to myself immediately, a surge of negative emotion can turn into a depression that lasts a couple days.

More and more, though, I'm able to work my way out of the flood using various strategies. The emotions can hit so hard that I'm often forced to stop what I'm doing and work on them.

I usually start by naming what's happening: that my surface mind is overreacting and having a dysregulated emotional response. I tell myself that I'm actually okay and can handle whatever has caused the reaction. I remind myself that what has upset me isn't actually that important—and certainly not worth the pain it's causing.

I often take three **deep breaths**, which is what my dear friend Nina always tells me to do.

I try to step back into another, bigger part of myself that can observe the part of me that's so upset. I try to align with that **observer** part of myself **to get some distance from the emotionally flooded part.**

This reminds me that I'm more than my overwhelming feelings.

I remember that I want to accept whatever it is that has upset me and that I can't control other people, places, and things. I remember that I'd rather be happy than be right (in cases that involve an argument).

I remind myself that I don't always feel the way I'm feeling then.

Sometimes, I write down what just happened and/or some affirmative statements emphasizing that I am okay and safe.

Doing some fast physical exercise for even a few minutes (whatever that is for you where you are: up and down stairs, jumping jacks, an exercise machine, a run, etc.,) can really get the emotions moving out. **I also ask for help: I close my eyes and ask the Universe to help me let this go.**

Calling or texting someone who understands can really help. For me, it's often my friend Marin, who reminds me to do the things I've just written here. Just being able to talk about it with her creates some distance between the overwhelming emotions and the rest of me.

Emotional dysregulation seems to me to be in keeping with my inner hyperactivity, aka hyperarousal: my very excitable nervous system. I don't only get irritated or angry fast, I also get emotionally excited and enthusiastic fast—about ideas, people, or places I encounter.

Bouts of emotional dysregulation affect each of us differently depending on our constitutions and background. If you have difficult stuff from childhood, or adult trauma, working on excavating those things with a therapist (talking therapist) can help you move through bouts of emotional dysregulation faster.

As always, awareness is the start.

Procrastination

Procrastination. Wow! Procrastination is like the catch-all problem where every challenging ADHD trait comes to party! I say this jokingly, but it's no joke.

When I'm off the beam, so much of what I want or need to do has a layer of resistance around it, like an invisible wall.

Breaking through that wall of resistance can be a bewildering, discouraging struggle (why the f*ck can't I just do this?). And when I don't have any compensating strategies in place to break through the wall, I walk away: I put the thing off: I don't do it.

And, once I don't do it, **the task gets shoved into another dimension—somewhere in the back of my mind**—which makes it much harder to find in the future. And voila, procrastination!

We know that the ADHD brain is wildly turned on by what it's interested in but has a brutal time manufacturing the **motivation to do things it has no interest in.** There is science behind this—a lack of neurotransmitters for one—but **it is one of the most misunderstood and ridiculed parts of having ADHD. Ignorant people say, "Yeah, I don't like doing the dishes either, but I just do them."**

And although our **biology-based difficulty at becoming adequately motivated** to do things we aren't interested in is a big part of why we procrastinate, it's not the only reason.

Tug on almost any thread that makes up the ADHD tapestry, and it'll lead to procrastination issues.

Take my love of novelty, for instance. I've seen myself procrastinate on something I really need to do because **I'm busy going after some new and exciting thing in the moment** that has just popped into my mind.

And there are other underlying tendencies that contribute to procrastinating.

Take **indecision**: There may be a number of things that have to be decided (that I might not even be conscious of) before I can undertake a particular task. And these undecided issues repel me (energetically) and cause me to completely avoid even thinking about doing whatever it is that I'm putting off!

The ADHD **difficulty with organizing** and being able to break down a project into the actionable steps (aka sequencing or chunking) needed to complete it also easily leads to avoidance and procrastination.

Where I'll see the big picture of what needs doing to get a particular task done, **I don't as easily see where I should start work on it. So, I avoid the thing.**

Emotional issues, too, absolutely come into play and cause procrastination.

I procrastinate returning phone calls or initiating them. Sometimes it's because I don't want to deal with emotional issues concerning the person. But most of the time it's because **I want to avoid feeling socially awkward on the phone.** I interrupt a lot and I feel uncomfortable in silences and sometimes rush to say anything to fill them. I just don't like phone calls except with my closest friends who understand how I am on the phone.

Sometimes I procrastinate because **I'm emotionally tired** and don't have any initiating-type energy left in my tank—that day. Same when I'm overwhelmed by too many things on my mind. That blocks my energy and stops me from doing anything.

Finding adequate motivation to do things we don't want to do is a core ADHD pursuit. **Many of the entries in Part IV contain strategies for compensating for a lack of motivation.** Often, if we can just get started on something, we can get into it.

The good news is that once you begin supporting yourself in various ways, your whole self will get ever so slightly easier to handle and your tendency to procrastinate will lessen.

Rejection Sensitive Dysphoria

Relationships. Oh, man!

As my beautiful therapist Alison has said a couple times, "Relationships are hard!" And they're high stakes, too, I always think, because (in many deep and profound ways) we all need each other.

So, of course things don't go smoothly all the time. It's nothing new to me to recognize the pain people can and do go through when they experience rejection. It can be absolutely devastating.

But what is new to me is therapists and mental health workers talking about and researching a new grouping of symptoms they're calling rejection sensitive dysphoria (RSD).

According to a study published in the June 2007 issue of the Journal of Cognitive Neuroscience, rejection sensitivity is **"the tendency to anxiously expect, readily perceive, and intensely react to rejection."**

Think about that: "to expect, readily perceive, and intensely react to rejection."

I mention RSD here because I think many women with ADHD have some RSD. I believe that we were either born with it or developed it living in a society that has made us feel like we don't fit in. Or both.

Some women suffering from a bout of RSD actually expect to be criticized or otherwise rejected (to different extents). Other times they're just highly sensitive to perceived rejection.

An expectation of rejection taints your way of perceiving other people's actions, causing you to feel wildly rejected and hurt by even the slightest hint of criticism you detect in someone else.

Because the brain's reactions to rejection are heightened, often a perceived rejection isn't even real!

I can think of times I felt rejected by something as insignificant as a stranger not saying hello at a party! Plenty of perceived slights are so often not directed at you at all. Generally, people are just wrapped up in their own stuff and oblivious to you.

But the pain—which activates the same parts of the brain that become activated when we are hurt physically—is real.

When something is painful, the mind starts looking for ways to ensure that we never experience it again: Women may **withdraw from social situations**, become **anxious about encounters**, or **stop participating in activities** to avoid the possibility that they'll end up in pain—**embarrassed, ashamed, or hurt.**

No matter what RSD is called or how it's categorized, clearly some people are more sensitive to rejection than others.

If you're a woman with ADHD and are highly sensitive to rejection—and some experts believe RSD is either part of ADHD or co-occurs with ADHD to a significant degree—it's a hugely helpful dynamic to become aware of so you can start to get some help with it.

I'm sure I'm somewhat rejection sensitive. But I've done a lot of work on myself for a long time—on my ADHD, in therapy, 12-step programs, and more—that has given me various psychological and behavioral tools to help maneuver through bouts of thinking I'm being rejected—or when, indeed, I am rejected!

If you recognize RSD in your life, you can start giving it your attention.

Losing Interest/Fickleness

Depending on the day, I might hotly declare that ADHD is a colossal pain in my ass OR that I'm grateful to have this unusual mind and all the awarenesses it allows me!

I change my mind a lot. I can love something Tuesday and be entirely indifferent to it by the week's end.

An ADHDer's interests are deep and wide and attracted to what's new. I've abandoned all sorts of people, persuits, and things because I'll suddenly really want something new and different.

On the other hand, there are experts who believe that this ADHD trait is responsible for much of mankind's forward progress: Many believe that in primitive societies, it was the ADHDers whose desire to explore and forge into new territories led to colossal discoveries, inventions, and new lands. (Meanwhile, neurotypicals were equally required to put down roots and keep the home fires burning, so to speak.)

This is a powerful ADHD asset that can also be hard to manage if you don't have any useful strategies on hand.

For instance: I'd been consistently writing this book, with great excitement, for a couple months and then boom, two weeks ago, I stopped.

Why? I'd lost all interest in it.

But now, a couple weeks later, I'm back to writing it again. For whatever reason, I seem to have endless things to say about ADHD. And I've taken that as a sign that I should stick with the book.

And, because I've worked with so many ADHD strategies, I could recognize where I was at, psychologically, and pick the right tool to use to position myself to re-approach the book.

And that tool is the comforting "every little bit counts" strategy: I'm only asking myself to write on the book for one hour a day.

That's all. No matter whether the writing is good, bad, or the worst ever. One hour a day.

Sensory Processing Sensitivity

I'd never heard of Sensory Processing Sensitivity (SPS) until I mentioned on Instagram the agony I felt shopping at T.J. Maxx one day, and a lot of women commented.

It's taken me all these years to really acknowledge how sensitive I am and to learn that being a Highly Sensitive Person (HSP) is a real thing.

I think many women with ADHD are highly sensitive people and have SPS.

My impression is that women with Sensory Processing Sensitivity have highly calibrated sensory apparatuses that experience everything more strongly than the average person. And it's more than the feeling of just having to rip off your bra the second you get home, but it's like that. Lights that don't bother anyone else can be distractingly too bright for you; tags on clothing can be as intolerable as a bra; loud noise can highjack your attention; somebody wearing too much perfume can drive you from a room.

Sensitive ADHDers have highly calibrated central nervous systems that receive sensory input more strongly than most neurotypical nervous systems.

But it's not only that. We also tend to have deeper cognitive experiences of *everything, good and bad*. Which means we think a lot—for longer and more deeply—about almost everything.

Consequently, something that may just be irritating or easily ignored for other people can become incredibly distracting or distressing to someone with SPS.

Before I knew anything about SPS, I used to make fun of myself as being like the princess in the fairy tale *The Princess and Pea* who could feel a single pea under a tall pile of mattresses.

Big stores are especially hard. I usually feel really anxious in them, continually whispering to myself, "I gotta get out of here, I gotta get out of here." The whole environment in T.J. Maxx wipes me out: the lights, the noise, even the air (and it isn't just off-fuming from the chemicals used in manufacturing).

I get spacey as my energy gets shattered by these subtle assaults. My poor brain, through my eyes, takes in thousands of items at a glance that all try to grab my attention.

As is so often the case with ADHD challenges, being highly sensitive is also the root of tremendous creativity.

Word.

Now and Not Now: Time Myopia

I love massages, but they cost a lot, so I only get one every once in a while when it suddenly hits me that I'm absolutely dying for one.

At those times, I call all over *trying to find an opening for right then* but, usually, there's nothing available that day. And the masseuses will always say **they can schedule me for the next day or the next, but I almost never make the appointment.**

But when the next day comes, I wish I'd made it!

I've learned that the reason I don't make an appointment for another day is because *I can't actually imagine that a future date will come when a future me will be really happy to have a massage appointment.*

No: Deep down, I feel that if I don't get the massage right then, it won't exist. Some people say that ADHders perceive only two times: **Now and not now.**

I'm strongly attracted to the present moment. All I can do right NOW feels real and alive and right. Having to schedule anything for later stops me in my tracks.

This stems from an ADHD cocktail of traits. First among them for me is a hard-to-explain inability to imagine, know, or feel that something scheduled for a future time *will be real.*

Something scheduled for a future time has very little juice for me. It's as though something planned is grayed-out and unavailable.

It's Now or Never for me with so many things.

This strong bias for the here and now contributes to a bunch of difficult, as well as constructive, behaviors.

For instance, the **Now or Never perception makes it hard to decide what to do first** when confronted with a list of things I need to do: I always want to do everything first, right that minute.

But you can't do everything first! We live in linear time, so one thing has to come after the other. A neurotypical person needing to choose what to do wouldn't be burdened by an unconscious desire to do everything NOW. A neurotypical mind would, ideally, prioritize what to do first and second and third, etc., and tackle things one by one, over time.

On the other hand, my Now or Never energy has driven me to go after things spontaneously that have come into my mind in the here and now and led me to some great things. Like writing this book. Like learning the basics of music theory in one night and starting to learn how to play the guitar. Like beginning to learn the craft of writing because I just had to communicate something that happened to me that day.

Obviously, the juice we find in the new and the now also causes us to be easily seduced by a passing thing or thought. You know: When you walk into a room to get your computer charger and end up repotting a plant.

All of this is part of what many refer to **as time myopia or time blindness**. Usually, it results in a lot of us being late for things—unable to judge how much time something will take.

Really interesting, right?

Overwhelm

For me, feeling overwhelmed is a background anxiety that everything is one big, intertwined jumble of loose ends that I can never tie up: things, relationships, obligations, chipped paint, passions, desires, objects, thoughts, vitamins, dreams, laundry, PMS, going gray, giving birth, cleaning, cooking, eating, clothing, budgeting, communicating, exercising.

I'm convinced that a large part of why women with ADHD feel even more overwhelmed than the average multi-tasking, cell phone-controlled neurotypical woman is because of their wide-open awareness of so much—and the feeling that they have to do something about, with, to, or for all these awarenesses/things/ideas/options.

Tendencies to be unorganized, inspired, impulsive, attracted to something new, indecisive, and restless also make it extremely difficult to keep things orderly in a world that demands so much from each of us.

There are many ways to unload your full plate and ease the chaos when you feel you have too much to take care of and don't know where to start, or how you're going to handle your life. Many of these suggestions can be found in the entries in Parts III and IV of this book.

And remember that whatever small move you make to ease any of your challenging ADHD traits will relieve, even if only ever so slightly, bit by bit, your feelings of being overwhelmed.

What ADHD is, Officially

ADHD stands for Attention Deficit Hyperactivity Disorder, which, according to the National Institute of Mental Health, is a "disorder marked by an ongoing pattern of inattention and/or hyperactivity-impulsivity that interferes with functioning or development."

Some people call it ADD (attention deficit disorder) but the proper medical term is ADHD. There is widespread dislike for this term for two main reasons: For one, ADHD doesn't always cause a deficit of attention as the name would imply, but instead affects a person's ability to direct, sustain, and regulate their attention (or focus). And second, not everyone with ADHD is hyperactive!

The medical party line about ADHD is contained in the Diagnostic and Statistical Manual of Mental Disorders, aka the DSM-5 (the fifth edition). It's the book used by mental health professionals to diagnose mental disorders worldwide.

The DSM-5 divides ADHD into three subtypes: predominantly inattentive; predominantly hyperactive/impulsive; and a combination of the two.

Under each of the first two types, the DSM-5 lists nine criteria used to diagnose the disorder. To be diagnosed as the inattentive subtype or the hyperactive/impulsive subtype, you would need to experience six of the nine criteria for at least six months. (ADHD symptoms can be inconsistent and come and go in degrees. Not only that, but all people experience traits that people with ADHD experience, but to a much lesser degree. It's the frequency and intensity of the symptoms and how long you're bothered by them that is critical to diagnosis.)

To be the combo type, you'd need to experience six of the nine criteria in each of the two types for at least six months.

These, again, are just guidelines to help therapists and mental health clinicians when making a diagnosis.

Most people think of women with ADHD as the hyperactive/impulsive type: a multitasking, talkative, intuitive, high-energy woman with a million things going on. The inattentive type's traits are harder to spot: They can be quiet, vague, and dreamy, often deep in their own world. The combination type is someone with traits from both sub-types and can present as anything!

For all these reasons, ADHD is called a spectrum disorder—there are many, many parts to it, and some people have some parts and not others.

Sadly, Western medicine positions itself to treat disease rather than enhance wellness, so the DSM doesn't list the positive aspects of ADHD, even though they're so readily recognizable they could be used as additional criteria!

Lastly, different people have a harder time with ADHD than others. But most can do well—with help.

Which is what this book is all about.

PART II

She What?#!: Essential ADHD Assets

The entries in this section explore the assets of the ADHD mind and how they sometimes feel.

The Orchid Hypothesis

> "We've just coined a term: 'Recognition Sensitive Euphoria,'... which refers to our [ADHDer's] enhanced ability to make constructive use of praise, affirmation and encouragement. As much as we can get down in the dumps over a minute criticism, **we can fly high and put to great use even small bits of encouragement or recognition.**"
>
> —From "ADHD 2.0," by Edward M. Hallowell, M.D., and John J. Ratey, M.D.

Long before I knew anything about ADHD, I recognized that **I do much better if I get some form of helpful support from almost anyone, with almost anything.**

If I just have someone involved in a task with me (even if it's just through talking about it), I can usually get motivated more easily. Often, I end up doing a great job at something I might not otherwise have had the motivation to begin.

Turns out, researchers have uncovered some science explaining my constructive response to support.

A new-ish hypothesis holds that **people with ADHD** (and other neurodiversities) **have a genetic predisposition to excel beyond the average neurotypical at various endeavors *when in a nurturing environment.*** Known as the **Orchid Hypothesis**, it likens ADHDers to orchids—plants that will blossom in a dazzling array of shapes and colors, that far outlast any other flower, *when they are cared for well.*

The theory holds that the same genes that allow us to thrive in positive environments also cause us to fare less well in stressful ones—neglect, abuse, criticism, lack of love.

In other words, the genetic markers for ADHD give a person a much greater sensitivity and response to being both neglected and nurtured.

In the book *The Orchid and the Dandelion*, W. Thomas Boyce, M.D., likens neurotypical people to **dandelions**, hardy flowers that can thrive in even rugged conditions. **Orchids**, on the other hand, will only blossom if well cared for.

These ideas are examples of how nature and nurture work together: Genetics positions us with the potential for various traits and the environment shapes how they unfold.

The same ultra-sensitivity that causes women with ADHD to wither in hostile or careless environments, allows us to soar beyond the average neurotypical in supportive circumstances.

The journalist David Dobbs outlines the hypothesis in a fascinating article in the December 2009 issue of *The Atlantic* entitled "The Science of Success."

All of which is to say that we ADHDers have deep reserves of resilience, creativity, strength, enthusiasm, and all-around power.

These are gifts worth protecting and excavating. *Remember this.*

Being Highly Creative and Imaginative

"Imagination is more important than knowledge. For knowledge is limited to all we now know and understand, while imagination embraces the entire world, and all there ever will be to know and understand."

—Albert Einstein

"A running joke that my best friend and I have had since we were twelve or thirteen has been I am the one who comes up with the idea, and she is the one who organizes and implements it—usually in reference to us taking over the world when we were younger, now it's just any plan. **I'm the ideas person and she's the logistics person.** I always knew myself well enough to know that follow through on a plan was not something I would do because it would be too overwhelming, but I had always just chalked it up to laziness because I didn't have any other words for it (before getting diagnosed). I'm really lucky to have met her at such a young age, and to still have her as a friend."

—Jessica, diagnosed at 31, when the pandemic eliminated "all the structure I'd unconsciously built for myself."

Over and over, I keep reading how the same traits that can challenge an ADHDer also give her enhanced creative tendencies.

Scientists who study the keys to creativity have identified the traits of highly creative people to learn how to promote outside the box thinking and fuel invention and discovery.

These characteristics include being spontaneous, novelty-loving, risk-taking, energetic, curious, unconventional, impulsive, and hyperactive.

Most of these characteristics are ADHD traits. So, yes: **The very same traits that can be so difficult to handle can also be the source of great imagination and creativity.**

One facet of the ADHD brain responsible for its enhanced imagination and creativity is its strength at something known as *divergent thinking. This is the ability to spin off many ideas from a single starting point.*

The following is an example of how divergent thinking might play out in everyday life.

Say you're in a group meeting of some sort trying to solve a problem.

The accepted, unspoken, conventional methodology will be to take a step-by-step, linear approach, trying to sort out the problem by examining one aspect of it at a time, in order.

But, that's not an ADHDer's natural approach! We're much more likely to jump right into the middle of a problem, grasping the issue as a whole, and start working away at it in many directions at once! And even though we may be excitedly hatching clusters of possible solutions, the group is unlikely to be able to follow our leads because they need to maintain an orderly approach and we seem to them to be all *over the place!*

This is one of the ways ADHDers can be wildly misunderstood and also a good example of our advanced potential to spin off dozens of ideas from a single starting point, aka, to think divergently. What an asset!

This all-directions-at-once, non-linear, big-picture problem solving style is also known as **lateral thinking.**

In a purely creative environment—say, a room full of app designers, schoolchildren, creative directors, copywriters, or any other group working on an issue—ADHDers will likely be responsible for many of the best ideas.

The hope is that as society becomes more educated about how our neurodivergent brains operate, people will expand their awareness of all the ways intelligence can be communicated.

When and where that happens, or is happening, we will all have learned to understand each others' styles of thinking, working, and problem solving and be richer for it: Neurotypical and Neurodivergent alike!

Being Highly Intuitive

"I love knowing my innate wisdom and creativity give me everything I need to flourish as an ADHDer."

—Gabi, (IG: @gabi_fisher)

Intuition is a way of coming to know something without reasoning it out consciously. All people are intuitive, but women in general are known for their stronger intuitive powers—and women with ADHD are even more intuitive.

Most agree that intuition relies largely on the **ability to make unconscious connections among many sources and to see patterns where others don't.**

Part of an ADHDer's highly functioning intuition stems from our natural ability to notice so much all the time. The same wide-open awareness that can cause us to be attracted to and distracted by every passing thing, also gives us a large palette of information.

In other words, because the ADHD mind regularly takes in a massive volume of input, it has an enormous storehouse of information for the unconscious to work with.

Experts say that most people with ADHD are often more interested in **how things connect** than the things themselves!

We're often curious about what's going on *behind the scenes*. Whereas a neurotypical woman will likely be content with the surface enticements of any given scenario, **my wide-open curiosity** will want to know why the cafe chose to group the outdoor tables where they did, which method of coffee-making my friend used, or how someone names and organizes their computer documents.

With so much sensory input available to a mind fascinated by how things connect, it's no wonder the ADHD mind is highly intuitive.

Before I learned about ADHD—before I knew I had it—I just went with whatever came up in life. I wasn't a planner, I didn't set goals, I didn't prioritize, I didn't even make simple pros and cons lists. I now know I could have done so much better if I'd known about my ADHD and learned some helping strategies.

And although I lost a lot of opportunities and stumbled around quite a bit, I know now that I did as well as I did because I have highly evolved intuition that can often see the whole picture.

I bet you can, too.

Having the Ability to Hyperfocus

Years ago, before I knew anything about ADHD, I was confused when my friend told me that her husband had ADHD. I knew him to be enthusiastic in conversation—interested in all kinds of things and typically flitting from subject to subject, which of course *I love*. What confused me was that he also regularly got so deeply into his work—he's a watchmaker—that he would be in his workshop lost to the world for hours and hours.

At that time, I'd assumed that people with ADHD weren't able to pay attention well, as the name Attention Deficit Hyperactivity Disorder makes you think.

Much later, I learned that the name is misleading (and highly disliked by experts), and that **it isn't that ADHDers lack attention but that our ability to *deploy our attention on demand* is irregular.**

Difficulty deploying our attention results in the terribly frustrating and confounding ADHD trait of being unable to get motivated to do things we're not interested in—one of ADHD's most difficult challenges.

And yet that same energy can also swing to the opposite pole allowing us to become so motivated and deeply attentive that *we flip into hyperfocus!*

So, hyperfocus is another example of how difficult traits can also be wielded to productive and positive ends.

Hyperfocus generally kicks in when you're doing something you naturally like. I think of it as similar to what athletes call peak experiences, wherein they're totally absorbed in the game, playing so deeply hard and fast that everything else fades away. It's a powerful force.

Working hand in hand with other ADHD assets, like a fertile imagination, hyperfocus can take unique ideas and transform them into 3D creations!

My best times of being hyper-focused are when I'm writing, and I'm so in the groove that every time I glance at the clock a few hours have gone by. I love the feeling.

Do you recognize it in yourself?

The Ability to Have Laser Focus Under Pressure

It's so interesting that a significant number of emergency room doctors and firefighters have ADHD.

Unlike the neurotypical brain that gets understandably nervous and overloaded in an emergency, the ADHD brain is calmed by the strict demands of an emergency. **The critical importance of attending to an emergency vanquishes any other distractions and occupies the ADHD brain fully, allowing it to focus with laser-like precision.**

When everybody else is freaking out, ADHDers can take control in fast and effective ways.

Emergencies stimulate the ADHD brain, and our whole remarkable head apparatus lights up (like Bradley Cooper in the movie *Limitless*).

Laser focus is a form of hyperfocus, but worth recognizing as a distinct asset.

Other pressure situations, like deadlines, can have a similar effect on our brains. Say, doing your taxes on April 14. Or, in my case, having a story due to an editor. Knowing that I absolutely have to meet a deadline somehow frees me to let go of all the other things on my mind, and focus fully on a story.

Stressful and serious pressure situations silence the mental-emotional constellation of background distractions that live in your mind.

When there's a pressure situation upon you, all the other stuff that usually grabs your attention gets grayed out.

What a relief! And what an asset!

Being Improvisational, Resourceful, and Inventive

> *"I taught myself how to do a lot of fixing of machinery while I worked at a pharmacy in high school because it was a nightmare to work without it and I am not very good at working inefficiently: I get so frustrated when I'm forced to do things slowly.*
>
> *So I taught myself how to fix things like the computers, registers, and the medication counting machine, or would ask the IT guy how he fixed them so I could do it next time and he wouldn't have to drive up from his home office four hours south. I remember walking in multiple times, when I was on late shift, and being told the med counting machine had been broken all morning and having it up and running again within a few minutes."*
>
> —Jessica, 32

Jessica obviously has an affinity for mechanics, which not everybody has, but I think a lot of us have the resourcefulness that she used to fix broken things at her workplace.

I like to fix stuff—or find work-arounds—too.

I think of myself as being kind of like this small junk drawer I have in my kitchen. It's a jumble, but I can always seem to find just the right thing in there that I need.

When something breaks or a problem arises, I can pretty much, within reason, of course, find a way around it and come up with (invent) a substitute. I can improvise.

Being resourceful and good at improvisation may sound a lot like being imaginative and creative, and they do often all work together. But they're distinct talents, and it's important to point them out. If we don't, we might miss recognizing them in ourselves.

One of the key traits that makes ADHDers so terrifically resourceful and improvisational is our tendency to operate slightly outside the conventions of society. It's not that we're rule breakers consciously, it's just that we're habituated to perceiving people, places, and things from a slightly eccentric angle. Because of this, **our thinking is less bound to the conventional purpose of a particular thing and our inner vision has fewer filters.** This makes it easier to see how we might be able to use something that, as a rule, is supposed to be confined to one particular purpose!

This ability to see objects in a larger context than their commonplace frames and find solutions in their parts (that others overlook) is one of the keys to being ingenious, inventive, and resourceful. And, **in circles where experts study invention, it is a highly prized trait known as *conceptual expansion.***

There's just a lot on tap in the ADHD head and thus a lot for minds to work with when problem solving. The same excess of thoughts that is so distracting much of the time also gives rise to ingenious solutions.

ADHDers' abilities to see the big picture comes into play here, too. Whereas a neurotypical brain approaches issues in a logical, ordered way, the ADHD brain has a less linear point of view. We somehow perceive an issue whole, grasping all parts of the thing at once.

ADHDers also see patterns, you know? Where others see chaos, the ADHDer can often discern patterns that connect. That feeds the ability to improvise and find resources where others can't.

And then there's the ADHDer's love of novelty and learning. This love fuels the desire to try this, that, and the other thing! So, there's energy and focus behind the desire to improvise solutions.

When a problem arises, I'd trust a woman with ADHD to come up with some ingenious workaround. She can usually pull something original out of nothing, improvise fluidly, and work fast to make new connections between and among things while repurposing objects to fit together in new ways.

Boom!

Having the Ability to Heal

> *"Nobody escapes being wounded. We are all wounded people, whether physically, emotionally, mentally, or spiritually. The main question is not 'How can we hide our wounds?' so we don't have to be embarrassed, but 'How can we put our woundedness in the service of others?' When our wounds cease to be a source of shame, and become a source of healing, we have become wounded healers."*
>
> —Henri J. M. Nouwen

I deeply believe in the above quote. It seems to me that everybody's got something, not just those of us with ADHD.

And I'm not saying this makes your struggles any less real. God knows, I've shed a lot of tears in my life, and still do. But something constructive can come from our pain.

Years of grappling with difficult ADHD traits makes you a kind of expert on them.

So, if you're willing, you can share your experience with people you encounter and help them.

At this point, I'm totally open about my issues because I know that millions of people are struggling with ADHD, depression, emotional dysregulation, addiction, and other mental/emotional/

neurobiological disorders or conditions. Either that or they have a loved one who is.

So I share about it: at grocery stores, hair salons, cafes, dinners out, parties, chance encounters, anywhere: I'm open about it if it comes up.

There's just way too much shame out there in the world about this stuff, and I have to do what I can to get free of it.

And it always makes me feel good to see the look of awakening on peoples' faces when something dawns on them as they register one thing or another.

Sometimes it's shock that a somewhat-normal-acting person like me has mental illness (depression) and a disorder, ADHD. Sometimes it's a connecting of the dots that makes them realize that their friend, child, sibling, or neighbor must have ADHD. And sometimes it's that they themselves have been struggling in silence and ignorance about one of these conditions and that maybe they don't have to bear it alone anymore.

The whole world needs healing, and humans have the capacity to heal. **Connecting with each other about our challenges and pain is a healing act.**

We who have ADHD have the opportunity to be healers and that's a noble calling: a path with purpose.

How about that?!

Being a Catalyst

A lot of the time, I find myself somewhere wanting to rave to a sales clerk, barista, or group of people something about the situation we're in that sets it in a bigger context than the real, 3-D situation we're in.

At a neighborhood meeting, say, instead of thinking about the problem, I'll be marveling at all the events that had to have come together to deliver each of us to this same block. Or how unbelievable it is that our brains can identify each new face as distinct from the trillions of faces that have ever been!

A similar thing happened the other day at the farmer's market. I was chatting with a potter about a bowl she'd made that got me thinking about all the clay bowls excavated from archeological sites all over the world going back millennia.

When I suggested that she advertise her booth with an image of an earthenware bowl from ancient Egypt, she loved the idea.

Often when I mention something like this, people glance at me and don't say a thing.

Other times, though, what I say will pique someone's interest—like it did with this potter—and it'll spark the other person to think of an issue in a new way.

Although this *divergent thinking* can be challenging for women with ADHD, it can also be the source of eccentric perspectives that catalyze others' thinking toward creative ends.

The ability to reimagine issues outside their conventional frames creates unusual points of view—ideas, observations, questions, suggestions, reflections—that ultimately fuel innovation, evolution, and progress.

This is very cool to me because I know that diversity in an ecosystem gives it great resilience and fertility, and I think that principle applies here to the "ecosystem," that is the collective mind in which we exist.

By injecting alternate awarenesses into our collective conversation, ADHDers fertilize human thought, helping move things forward.

Being Highly Empathetic

*"Sing the songs you still can sing.
Forget your perfect offering.
There is a crack in everything.
That's how the light gets in."*

—Leonard Cohen

"I think of myself as very compassionate. I am very connected to people. I can feel people's pain before they even express it. I always end up talking to people who are hurting—if they're open.

I allow them to share what's going on. I try not to be a fixer but I try to be a sounding board so they can get things off their chest. I try to be understanding. I'm not judgmental. People have their own situations that they're going through and I'm not going to judge.

Literally, I do this with strangers. I'll be sitting at Starbucks and see someone that's down and I'll say, are you ok? I'm just there to say, I get you, tell me about it and I can help you work through it. Or I can just listen.

It's a balance because it can be very heavy so sometimes it can be overwhelming. But I know they need it at that moment. And if people say they're okay, I will walk away.

But, often I get, 'Oh my gosh I don't know why I'm telling you all of this!'"

—Yakini, ADHDer, entrepreneur, and mother of two

Because women with ADHD attach to the world at a slightly different angle (dance to a different drummer), **we're intimately acquainted with the discomfort of being perceived by others as different. And the awareness of this "*crack*" in ourselves often gives us a natural awareness of and compassion for others who are different in any kind of way.**

Not only that, but because women with ADHD are highly **sensitive perceivers** they can feel and sense others' emotions more deeply than the average Joe *without even trying*.

All of which makes women with ADHD highly empathetic: You want to give money to a guy on the street, you notice the old person with a limp, you're crushed at the sight of abandoned pets, your heart aches when a friend is hurt, you champion those less fortunate than yourself and people on the edge.

Our empathy has a lot to offer the world.

Empathy is the gateway to peace: How can you battle someone whose pain you empathize with?

Empathy engenders understanding: When your heart is open, your mind opens.

Empathy builds bridges among us by showing that we all bleed the same, which gives us a feeling of being connected to each other beneath our surface differences.

Empathy is a great gift but it's worth mentioning that empathy can be a problem if you have other issues.

I know I used to give so much of myself to people whose emotional pain I sensed that it caused me to lose touch with my own needs and feelings.

This evolved from having grown up with a raging father.

To try to prevent him from exploding, I learned to track his feelings so I could ward off a fight. This nervous hyper vigilance became a real problem for me. All those years of feeling my father's feelings prevented me from feeling my own. It also trained me to vacate myself and track other people's feelings later in life. As an adult, I've done lots of work on this issue in therapy, Al Anon's Adult Children of Alcoholics, AA, and Marijuana Anonymous (MA).

But if your **boundaries** are good and you know who you are and what you feel, it can't be anything but beautiful and good to have empathy for others' pain.

And women with ADHD have it in spades.

Novelty-Loving

> *"I'm an adventurer. I control my whole family's novelty intake. Anytime we go on a day trip it's all me [who plans where we go and what we do]. Learning that I had ADHD made me stop resenting that role or seeing it as a gender thing—that I plan everything. It's me who's always looking for new things and I'm good at finding them. I have a love of pleasure and novelty and I want to share that with other people."*
>
> —Sarah, writer, child psychologist, and mother of two in the Bay Area

Like Sarah, I've got a love of novelty.

According to Dr. C. Robert Cloninger, an American psychiatrist who studies well-being, **novelty-seeking is one of the personality factors that can keep people happy and healthy.**

It's a simple thing to describe: I am attracted to—interested in, desirous of—things, ideas, and people—that are new or newly-occurring to me. **A love of novelty underlies curiosity. And curiosity propels us into the unknown.**

I love being around someone who's curious about things.

One curious person can lift the spirits of a whole group!

Novelty-loving brings us into the present moment. It elevates the proceedings, whatever they are, by whipping up some positive energy around them.

Researchers who study personality types in relation to how humankind evolves, believe that ADHDers descend from earlier humans who were novelty-lovers.

The theory holds that there had to be novelty-seekers so that early humans could find new horizons. On the other hand, there were also people who were novelty-averse. And those people were also needed to keep the home fires burning and maintain stability.

Great, right?

Being Fast Jugglers aka Multitaskers

"I worked in a very busy pharmacy for just under ten years, starting just after I got out of high school. When I worked there I did not know I was ADHD, but when I look back on it there are a lot of things I think are related to my ADHD, that were useful working in a very busy pharmacy.

I could listen to multiple things going on at once, so I used to listen to the names being given at the pick-up counters, so I could look them up and get them to the pharmacist before the cashier even noticed.

I used to get quite irritated because no one else in the pharmacy seemed to do this, or even pay attention to a couple things at a time, and I would be paying attention to the pickup counter, typing prescriptions, listening for the med counting machine bell (just in case it needed a refill), and possibly carrying on a conversation with a co-worker at the same time.

It never occurred to me that they just didn't have the capability of paying attention to more than one or two things at a time, that their brains didn't work the same way mine did until about two months ago when I was reminiscing with my best friend, who also worked there for a bit, about the chaos of working there.

One of my co-workers used to call me the hummingbird of the pharmacy because I was always moving around the place doing a little bit of everything at top speed."

—Jessica, 32

I know exactly what Jessica is talking about. I'm just like that.

I'm also aware that there are studies that prove that when people think they're multi-tasking, what they're really doing is switching rapidly from one awareness of something to another.

So, it occurred to me that what we fast heads are doing when we're doing what Jessica did at her pharmacy job is juggling—rapidly.

But whatever you call it, there's little doubt that women with ADHD are probably the best class of jugglers, aka multi-taskers, out there!

It's a very useful aspect of a fundamental trait of the ADHD brain: that wide-open focus that takes in so much all at once.

In contrast, our neurotypical friends naturally blur out much of what's going on outside their specific job. This allows them to maintain a calm, steady focus on whatever they're doing. I'm often soothed by my neurotypical friends' relaxed style of doing things but I'm essentially a multi-tasking juggler.

One style of doing things isn't better than another: All brains are good at some things and not good at other things. And other brains are good at other things and not good at other things.

Right?

PART III

The Approach/Getting Set Up

The entries in this section are about positioning yourself—physically, emotionally, psychologically, and spiritually—toward ADHD and the fact of your having ADHD. They also offer ways to situate yourself in various environments so you feel supported in a world that can hold you and your ADHD in a loving way.

Take a Battle Stance

God, do I love this woman, Ernestine Shepherd! She's 87 now (in 2023), and still holds the Guinness World Record she won in 2010 for being the oldest competitive female body builder.

She's inspired me since I saw a video of her talking about how she approaches each day.

She said she gets up at around 3 a.m., says her "devotions," eats the same high-protein meal every morning, then gets outside with a headband light on her forehead, and starts running.

And the part I remember the most is that she says she has to start singing loudly as she gets going, to psyche herself up.

She sings loud!

That's her battle cry. A cry to life that she's going to do this thing!

Ernestine's song is a psychic sword that cuts through her resistance.

This inspires me to acknowledge that a lot of life requires effort and hard work, not just ADHD.

And as the adorable writer Glennon Doyle says all the time, **"We can do hard things."**

Celebrate Neurodiversity

"I found test taking to be extremely difficult. It was not until graduate school that I accepted accommodations available for my ADHD. Really. I was preparing for my licensure exam. It was not the material I struggled with but managing my time during the test/quiz. The time restriction would increase my anxiety, making it more difficult to concentrate and retrieve the information that I needed to answer questions. I had a lot of difficulty in this one particular class. We would be given a quiz in the beginning of the class. Most of my classmates would finish quickly (and get good grades) and then begin to chat amongst themselves as others finished. This would be very distracting to me and also make me feel more anxious, rushed to finish my quiz and insecure that I was taking too long and the others would think I was not smart or holding up the rest of the class. **The accommodations I received allowed me extra time to complete tests and quizzes**. *This allowed me to take my time with each question and response, carefully consider my answer and not feel rushed or anxious during the exam. At times, I even took the quizzes in a quiet room by myself, which was also more helpful."*

—Julie

Thank God for all the focus on appreciating diversity out there now: the awareness around BLM, MeToo, LGBTQ, and, yes, neurodiversity.

The term *neurodivergent* applies to anyone with any kind of neurologically based difference like ADHD, autism, Asperger's, obsessive-compulsive disorder, auditory processing disorder, dyslexia, and more.

There's been so much shame around brain-based differences for so long. But now a lot of people are demanding that society recognize the value of neurodivergents' different ways of experiencing, interacting with, and processing the world.

Whole communities of neurodivergent people are out there connecting with each other—online and in person—including plenty of women with ADHD.

Advocates want societal recognition that their ADHD, for instance, is a natural variation in the human nervous system. This isn't to say that people with neurodivergent brains don't have challenges. We do.

That aside, society has to recognize that many of the challenges neurodivergent people encounter arise because our culture is designed to accommodate only neurotypical behavior.

By this, I mean that we're expected to express ourselves and interact with others according to a set of cultural expectations that govern the way society behaves.

For instance, we're supposed to approach issues in a step-by-step, orderly, one-after-the-other logical way. We're expected to be composed, amiable, stay on topic, and be cheerful—but not too cheerful.

Most neurodivergent people approach problem solving, work, relationships, and even simple conversation differently.

We want recognition that variations are normal and that people whose brains work differently are not broken but are an integral part of humanity, with rich contributions to make to society.

This starts with awareness and education. Once awareness grows, accommodations can be made at the institutional level: at schools, in workplaces, public meetings, and backyards.

Respecting neurodiverse people requires that society reevaluate how we recognize intelligence, seek solutions, and explore creativity.

The following are some ways we can accommodate people with various neurodivergencies:

- Offering flexible seating at work.
- Having quiet workspaces that limit distractions and/or allow telecommuting.
- Allowing earphones for those who concentrate best with music blasting.
- Offering flexible work schedules.
- Allowing a missed meeting when someone with time-blindness is hyperfocusing.
- Instituting some kind of play or exercise time at work to cultivate a free flow of ideas.

- Being open to tangential thoughts added to a conversation: avoiding knee-jerk rejections of stylistically unusual interjections.
- Following up oral instructions with written memos.
- Periodically holding slow, unstructured periods at meetings.

Women with ADHD can be leaders in the neurodivergent movement by educating others about neurodiversity. Sharing your needs with others will often start a cascade of awareness and action as your disclosures suddenly cause others to recognize what someone in their family or circle is going through.

And, because giving and receiving truly are one on a spiritual (unseen) level, you will benefit too, by this sharing. You'll feel useful. And that will make you feel connected and less alone. And your pride in yourself will blossom and this positive energy will ripple out across your life and into the world.

Uncover Self Love

"I don't need other people to be gentle with me for me to be gentle with myself, or to discover the systems that help me flourish as an ADHDer."

—Gabi, (IG: @gabi_fisher)

Gabi has beautifully embraced her ADHD and embodies the inherent value of neurodiversity. But many ADHDers still struggle with self acceptance and we're not alone: Many neurotypicals also struggle with self love.

Something to do with evolution and survival makes it easier for all people to dwell more on the negative than the positive. In any case, for whatever reason, **many of us live in what the great mindfulness teacher and therapist Tara Brach calls "a trance of unworthiness."** This means we walk around with a vague sense of guilt that we're not good enough, or we did something wrong, or we didn't do enough, or we're not enough, or we don't have enough.

And for women with ADHD, this shame that we're not enough can be even stronger. It evolves in girlhood from trying to fit into the dominant culture's step-by-step way of thinking and approaching things.

Anyway—working on self-love is the most important thing I do. I think all good things start with banishing shame and loving ourselves—simply because we exist.

There are many ways to work on this (see the entries in *Part IV* under *Self Care* and *Feelings*), but **I think the following exercise might help you *intellectually* understand that you're probably much more worthy of your own love than your mind tells you.**

(I know we have to work on shame on an emotional level, not intellectually, but having an intellectual understanding can buoy our commitment to working on our emotions.)

I propose that you think hard and write a list of the things you think of as your failures. By this I mean, list those parts of you that make you feel that you're unworthy of love: that you don't make dinner half the time, you're always forgetting things, you're moody, you lose important stuff, you yell at your kids, you're impatient, overwhelmed, messy, never finish anything.

After that list, make another: Think really deeply and list all the things you admire most in a human being.

Then, make a third list and **write down what you do like about yourself.**

As you look over the lists, I think you're going to find that you have many of the qualities that you most admire in another person and that the things that cause you to feel so badly about yourself are not very consequential.

I most admire people who treat all people equally, who have kind hearts, are honest, warm, open-minded, loving, compassionate, humble, courageous, enthusiastic, willing to change. That they can laugh at themselves.

Can you make a list of the things you admire about yourself?

I'll go first:

I really love people.

I believe that everybody is doing the best they can with what they have. (Nobody does things because they're trying to be disliked.)

I have a great sense of humor.

I always want to change myself for the better.

Even though I can be irritable and say sarcastic, mean things sometimes, I absolutely strive to be kinder all the time.

I know how to apologize.

I want to help others when I can.

I love new things and I'm enthusiastic about whatever I like.

I'm intuitive and pretty smart about people.

I love animals and they love me.

You?

Get Diagnosed

"So newly diagnosed I commenced research and had to agree. I have to say I cried. It was as if someone had removed all the negative labels I had piled on myself over the years. **To realize that I'm not stupid, careless, thoughtless, uncaring, lack commitment etc., etc., but it's that my brain works differently was wonderful.** *I began to see triumphs in previous 'failures.' Now I plan and strategize differently, planning for success. I also think back to my mum's behaviors and I'm sure she also had ADHD."*

—Erika, 65, mother of three

"I bought your 'Help for Women with ADHD' book yesterday on Amazon. It arrived today. I've read it all in one sitting and cried throughout the whole book. **For the first time in my life I feel understood and as if someone gets how my brain works. I'm so happy!"**

—Alaina, U.K.

The joke is that there's no 100 percent objective, put-your-money-on-it test that proves that a person has ADHD, like a blood test proves someone has diabetes.

According to experts, official **diagnoses can be made by** any one of a number of mental health professionals. These people can have any of the following titles: **psychiatrist, neurologist, psychologist, clinical social worker, or therapist.**

No matter which of these professionals you find, it's essential to determine if they specialize in ADHD, especially adult ADHD. That's what you're looking for.

Depending on who you go to, the person will take a long verbal history of you, detailing how you function, and have functioned, in the past. Their assessment may include various types of questionnaires and/or cognitive testing, and possibly a neuropsychological evaluation.

Getting diagnosed is so great, though, because only then can you orient yourself right and start getting support.

So many women I've heard from never got diagnosed as kids and only found out as adults. Every one of them was so relieved to know.

These days, since Covid ushered in virtual doctor's visits, many clinicians will meet virtually. This may be a possibility for you if you can't find anyone nearby.

Here are some things you can do right now to start looking for a professional who can assess and potentially diagnose you. (This is almost the same list that I've included in the entry "Try a Therapist at Least a Couple Times.")

- Check out the ton of information at the *Hallowell ADHD Centers*. The founder, Dr. Edward ("Ned") Hallowell, is a pioneer in the field of ADHD, has ADHD himself, and is a great champion of all ADHDers. He's the author or co-author of numerous books, including *Driven to Distraction*, and is arguably the most well-known speaker on ADHD in the western world. Hallowell has a number of centers across the U.S., including ones in New York City, the Boston area, California's Bay Area, and Seattle. And, with the advent of telehealth, you can connect with the centers from anywhere in the world.

Under *Services* on the main page of his site, you can click on *Diagnosis, Coaching, Medication, or Therapy* and under each find and fill out a short form to ask for a free (no pressure) *New Patient Consult* with one of the organization's clinicians (whose bios you can read on the site).

I can't think of a better place to start your quest to get diagnosed than the *Hallowell ADHD Centers*. I love Hallowell! (See the *Resources* section at the back of this book for a link to Hallowell's podcasts. He's also often a speaker at the annual, online, absolutely fabulous (and free!) *ADHD Women's Palooza*, which is also listed in the *Resources* section.)

- The *Psychologist Locator* is a tool created and maintained by the *American Psychological Association (APA)*. On the home page, fill in your area code or state and in the adjacent box, where it says *Practice Area*, write ADHD. That will get you a list of therapists who have a specialty in ADHD.

- Go to the *Psychology Today* website and enter your ZIP code or state. After a list of therapists comes up, click the *Issues* drop-down menu, and then *ADHD*.

- Go to the *ZenCare* website—at the bottom of this page is a long list of vetted ADHD specialists by state.

- **Terry Maitland, MSW,** is a psychotherapist, well-respected ADHD expert, coach, and author of the wonderful book, *Queen of Distraction*. Check out her site for help directing you to someone who can diagnose you. (Maitland is also almost always a speaker at the tremendously helpful and fabulous annual *ADHD Women's Palooza*, which is listed in the *Resources* section at the back of this book.)

Don't be afraid to cast your search far and wide. Be prepared with questions for the professionals you email or talk to. If you feel reluctant or shy, pretend you're a journalist doing research.

I suggest writing out what you're going to say and have it at the ready. Save it so you don't have to rewrite it every time you approach someone. If you have to leave a message, you could say something like the following:

"Hi. I'm just starting my search for someone who specializes in Attention Deficit Hyperactivity Disorder and who diagnoses it. I want to be evaluated to see if I have it. If you don't diagnose people yourself, can you recommend someone who does? I don't know much about this, but I'd really appreciate it if you have any help or ideas you can share with me. Thanks so much!"

Absolutely Consider Meds with an Experienced, Careful Prescriber

"Initially I was advised to go on medicine. **I take a stimulant called Elvanse. I can only say that it's changed my life.** *I suppose it's a success story for me because all those years I'd been so exhausted, constantly drained by the stress of this endless processing in my brain.*

It's really helped me. I can't emphasize enough how much it slows my brain down and the emotions that would just take me over in the past. I lost jobs I should have excelled at because I was so up and down emotionally.

It calms me down, but it also makes my head clearer and I'm able to process info and work at a pace that is manageable. I'm coherent, I don't forget things, I'm just so much more functional now."

—Sara, 37, executive assistant, from the U.K.

One of the first things many women do when they realize they have ADHD, is look into medication. Medicine doesn't work for everyone, **but for a majority of women it is life-changing** *if it is prescribed correctly (this is a big issue).*

If working well, ADHD meds can increase your ability to focus on and stick with the work you're doing over a prescribed period of time in a day. For many, many women, medication is nothing short of a total game changer.

The most widely used ADHD medications are stimulants that work in the moment: In other words, they don't have to build up in your system over time, the way many medications do, but work soon after you ingest them—like an aspirin or a sedative does.

Contrary to the effect you'd expect from a stimulant, these medications can calm an ADHD mind by helping different parts of it communicate with each other more easily. Meds can also lessen your distractibility while also increasing your impulse control. A properly timed and titrated dose of the right medicine can allow you to focus well and have fluid attention for hours at a time.

There's no doubt how helpful and healing the right medicine is for many women, so **don't let anyone make you feel ashamed for using it.**

But in order for it to work—and for you to even discover if it will work for you—it's best to have a patient, experienced prescriber who is very knowledgeable about ADHD medicines.

Dr. Charles Parker, author of *New ADHD Medication Rules: Brain Science & Common Sense*, says it's essential for the prescriber and the person with ADHD to work closely during the beginning of treatment. Together you identify how long you need the medicine to work, known as duration of effectiveness, or DOE. From there, the prescriber chooses a medication and starts you out on a low dosage.

The patient is then required to monitor her response day by day and report back to the prescriber in a week or two. Depending on how the patient says the medicine has worked, the prescriber can tweak the dosage.

There are many dosing possibilities since there are various strengths of all the major meds as well as both immediate release and extended-release versions.

Some people don't do well on an extended release (unable to sleep at night) and end up taking a lower-dose, immediate release medicine in the morning and another dose mid-day.

Being prescribed too much, too little, one with the wrong release factor for your needs, or taken at the wrong time won't work well for you. And what's so awful about this is that then you'll get the mistaken idea that ADHD medicine won't work for you.

Wherever possible, search for a prescriber who has experience with ADHD. I know this can be difficult in some places but the advent of telehealth has expanded the possibilities. The five organizations and websites listed in *Try A Therapist at Least a Couple Times*, on page 122, are good places to look for a prescriber. If it ends up that your primary care provider is your only option, by all means, go to him or her. But if possible, find the best expert you can who knows all about these medications.

This is such a big issue. So often I see people who aren't getting the meds they could use because the dose or type of medication is all wrong!

Well-Rounded Treatment Approach

I know it's hard to tell an ADHDer to get help since getting motivated to do things we don't want to do is a fundamental difficulty of ADHD itself!

But you can't treat ADHD well just by getting a fanny pack for your phone (although it is an extremely useful strategy for some!).

No: To set yourself up really well, you could do more. Many experts agree that building a well-rounded support system is the best way to position yourself.

You'll want to consider your mind, body, and spirit around the whole thing—so we're looking at addressing our emotions, our bodies, and our connections with others out there in the world.

A good support infrastructure will buffer your challenges, freeing up some of the time you'd normally lose to rescheduling, returning and overturning things and plans, racing to catch up, doing things you don't want to do, feeling remorse, and more.

It sounds like a lot, but if you do it a bit at a time and—very important—learn to ask for help, you can get the ball rolling.

Among the types of treatment you may pursue over time:

- **Increase Your Basic Healthy Living and Wellness**

    Eating well, exercising, sleeping, learning to calm yourself, taking time in nature, getting light… all these things help. (See *Increase General Wellness, Part III*.)

- **Find a Therapist**

    Even if you only go to a therapist for a few sessions, please give it a try. Depending on what you need, you can work with a therapist in different ways. You may want to use them as an ADHD coach, helping you assess your needs. Or, you may end up working with a therapist on an ongoing basis, like I do. (See *Try a Therapist at Least a Couple Times, Part III*, for what you can do right this minute to find a therapist.)

- **Find an ADHD Coach**

    There are more ADHD coaches available now than ever since the Covid pandemic has taken many things online. You can work with a therapist as a coach or find a certified ADHD coach who is not a therapist. She can help identify and prioritize your needs. From there, she can help you take the actions necessary to implement particular strategies, or efforts, that will help structure your life, one at a time. Coaches, and therapists acting as ADHD coaches, can help you identify and work on a range of practical life skills. And, since many neurodivergent nervous systems like ours excel with support, you can get a big bang for your buck with an ADHD coach or therapist acting as a coach. (See *Find an ADHD Coach, Part III.*)

- **Find an ADHD Buddy**

    Do you have a friend who has ADHD that you could buddy up with? Or, do you have a close friend who will be willing to learn about ADHD and be there if you pick up the phone when you need help? Having a pal with ADHD is a way to get coach-like help for fun and for free! Connecting with another person who shares your same issues is so uplifting! (See *Find an ADHD Buddy, Part III.*)

- **Give ADHD Medication a Chance**

    ADHD medication is a basic necessity for many women with ADHD. Please give yourself the chance to try it. To determine if it can help you, it's essential to find a prescriber who is experienced at finding the right type and dosage. This generally involves starting you off very low and customizing your medication over the course of a few visits. Yes, it may be difficult to find an experienced prescriber, but once you do, you'll have done yourself a great favor. (See *Absolutely Consider Meds with an Experienced, Careful Prescriber, Part III.*)

- **Find Ways to Connect with Others**

    We're social animals, all of us humans, ADHD or not, and we need to connect with others to feel good. There are so many ways we can connect. (See *Get Connected, Part III.*)

- **Help Someone Else**

    I believe that part of each person's basic hard wiring is a desire to help others. Use this innate part of yourself to get connected by considering ways you can give back to your community.

    We ADHDers have a lot to give the world, whether we believe it or not. ADHD makes us sensitive perceivers and naturally compassionate people aware of other peoples' needs.

    So say hello or lend a hand. It might be just the thing that person needs that day to not feel so alone. And, it will make you feel good, too.

    Often you just have to recognize something to start seeing it.

Try a Therapist at Least a Couple Times

There are at least three good reasons to get yourself into a therapist's office if you've just been diagnosed with ADHD or if you're having a hard time with your ADHD at a particular point in your life.

If you've just been diagnosed, **a therapist *knowledgeable about* ADHD can help you understand what it is and suggest ways you can start to get some support**. She can also help you process whatever feelings you're having about your diagnosis.

Another way a therapist can help is that **you could use the therapist as an ADHD coach.**

And a third way **a therapist can help you is if you have unexamined trauma or neglect from childhood—or adulthood.** Excavating your feelings about your past pain can lessen the pressure they cause you in the present and give you more energy to both manage your ADHD challenges and allow your assets to flourish.

Even if you just go to a therapist a couple of times, please do it. And don't let yourself get side-tracked trying to find the perfect one: Perfection doesn't exist!

Yes, some therapists will be a better fit for you—but **the most important part is to get started by just going.** If you find someone, but don't like them, find someone else. Don't worry about disappointing the therapist: They realize that smart people know how important it is to find a therapist who is a good fit for them. They want a good fit, too.

You may end up only going a few times. Or, you may realize you have emotional and psychological stuff to talk about and do some work on that with her.

However it goes, it's good to start the process as soon as you suspect you may have ADHD, or you've just been diagnosed.

A therapist can help you figure out what comes next and what steps you could be taking. A therapist will also validate what you've been feeling, which is something so many of us struggle with.

Many therapists now offer virtual therapy via Zoom. This could be good for you if you're in an area where you can't find a therapist experienced in ADHD to suit you.

The key is to get the ball rolling. Since procrastination is one of the hallmarks of ADHD, why not grab your notebook right now and search some of the resources listed below?

(This is nearly identical to the list of resources I've included in the Get Diagnosed entry.)

- Check out the ton of information at the ***Hallowell ADHD Centers.*** The founder, Dr. Edward ("Ned") Hallowell, is a pioneer in the field of ADHD, has ADHD himself, and is a great champion of all ADHDers. He's the author or co-author of numerous books, including *Driven to Distraction*, and is arguably the most well-known speaker on ADHD in the western world. Hallowell has a number of centers across the U.S., including those in New York City, the Boston area, California's Bay Area, and Seattle. And, with the advent of telehealth, you can connect with the center from anywhere in the world.

Under *services* on the main page of his site, you can click on *diagnosis, coaching, medication, or therapy* and under each find and fill out a short form to ask for a free (no pressure) *New Patient Consult* with one of the organization's clinicians (whose bios you can read on the site).

I can't think of a better place to start your quest to find a therapist. I love Hallowell! (See the *Resources* section at the back of this book for a link to Hallowell's podcasts. He's also often a speaker at the annual online, absolutely fabulous—and free—*ADHD Women's Palooza*, which is also listed in the *Resources* section.)

- **Psychology Today** The website for this magazine has an enormous directory of therapists. It's searchable by state. To have a look around, go to the main page and click on *Find a Therapist*.

- **Call your primary care doctor** and ask for a referral. Tell them you're looking for someone who specializes in ADHD.

- **Psychologist Locator** This tool was created and is maintained by the *American Psychological Association* (APA). The APA counts more than 121,000 educators, clinicians, consultants, researchers and students among its members, and this registry allows you to find a professional in your area quickly and easily.

- **Find a Psychologist** At *Find A Psychologist*, you can sort therapists by specialty, which is extremely useful when you're looking for someone who has experience with ADHD. The professionals on this registry are all licensed psychologists who have been verified by the National Register of Health Service Psychologists.
- **Go to the *Zencare* website.** At the bottom of the homepage is a list of vetted ADHD specialists by state.

Once you've got a list of therapists, call them and leave a message if they don't answer.

You might want to write down what you're going to say so you remember the key points. Something like this:

"Hi. I'm in the process of searching for a therapist who specializes in ADHD. I'm not sure how the whole thing works, but I know it's important to have a good fit with a particular therapist, and I hope you can help me. The best times to reach me are … (fill in the blank). My name is (fill in the blank), and my phone number is (fill in the blank). Thanks so much."

You can start work on this right now!

Create Structure Whenever Possible

"I was initially diagnosed with ADD in high school, however at the time I decided I did not want to rely on medication. I was able to get through high school and college without medication. I think the reason why I was able to manage without medication, was because I had a very busy schedule; I had school/classes, a part-time job, sports or extracurricular activities, and needed to do homework in between. I did not have time to procrastinate, I only had certain blocks of time for each activity. **When I have a day off with no plans or a large chunk of time with nothing specific to do, I am not productive.** I feel excited to accomplish things and I am motivated to get a lot of things done, but I end up wasting more time trying to figure out what to do first than actually doing something. **However, when I have limited time or need to adhere to a schedule, I am way more efficient.**"

—Julie, physical therapist

For a lot of us, a busy schedule is a helpful thing, like it was for Julie in high school. For others of us, it's like a nightmare of never catching up and being late for everything.

I'm a freelancer, so I have almost no structure except what I create. And although I'm initially resistant to scheduling things, I need some structure or I'd fly off the planet.

So I do things at set times each week, week in and week out, which helps me feel anchored and a bit more grounded than I would otherwise.

You can create some structure by **scheduling various repetitive tasks for the same time and day each week.** This way, you won't have to struggle deciding whether or when to go grocery shopping, you'll have the time set in stone. Doing the same things at the same times creates a rhythm: a balanced, habitual series of actions that flow together naturally. Rhythm keeps routine maintenance from piling up behind your back.

A simple rhythm would be cleaning the bathroom or doing the laundry on the same day (old school wisdom) every week.

So, too, would be meeting a friend for coffee on the same day, at the same time each week, every other week, or even just monthly, like on the first Saturday. I've found this to be so wonderful! (Connecting is so important and so easy to neglect doing.)

It'll probably be hard to stay with your commitment in the beginning (you could change your mind about it being a good idea!). But if you can imagine that committing to a set time for a particular weekly task could help you—and you choose to work with it—try to stick with it for a couple months.

By stick with it, I mean **nurture the effort by giving it an enhanced sense of importance in your mind and using just that one tool until it becomes a habit.** This is how I've had to work with each strategy I've implemented: one at a time, one day at a time, until the thing becomes automatic.

Here's an example: I have obligations every Sunday, Tuesday, and Wednesday. I know I'll be out of the house, and in a certain part of town, so I stack nearby errands around those appointments: the bank, the fish market, the grocery store. I keep track of what I'm doing when and where in my notebook (aka my desk notebook: See *Desk Notebook: Info Capture System, Part IV*), which keeps me on track.

This structure feels good and also makes it easier to decide how to schedule other activities in the spaces around the structured events.

A weekly rhythm cuts down on worry and distractions, too. When I notice something needs doing, I can pretty easily figure out when I will have time to take care of it.

It's simple to start. Just jot down your existing commitments with other people (those are probably the ones you keep most regularly)—classes, deadlines, social events. Think about where you'll be and how you'll feel—and what you can add on to do while you are wherever it is that you'll be.

Before you know it, you'll feel your daily and weekly rhythms supporting you in all kinds of ways.

Increase General Wellness

"During Covid, the Balance app [a meditation app] was free, so I said okay, I'll do that and I do about a 10-15 minute session with it in the morning and then, if the day is super busy or if I'm feeling really overwhelmed, I'll stop in the middle of the day and deep breathe and say, 'I'm okay. I'm okay,' or at night I'll do it, too. And I think, over time, meditation and deep breathing have made a difference. I'd say it's one of the bigger things that has helped me. It quiets down the bunnies in my head— I call them bunnies."

—Joanne, Calgary, Canada, mother of two, education assistant

A lot of people, when they get diagnosed with any kind of health issue, start wanting to take better care of themselves. You know: Eat better, exercise, cut down on alcohol and drugs, sleep well, spend time outdoors, and more.

I think the same goes for ADHD. Whatever you can do that's good for your general health will ultimately be helpful for your ADHD. (I think of this as the hip-bone's-connected-to-the-thigh-bone theory.)

Even though the (largely ignorant [sorry]) general public may not consider ADHD to be a "real" health condition, it absolutely is. No, it's not easily measurable like heart trouble, high blood pressure, or liver disease, but there is a growing body of scientific evidence on ADHD. It is not a failure of your will power, a figment of your imagination, or a psychiatric condition.

Among the most telling physical evidence is the fact that ADHD brains seem to be low in some brain chemicals (aka **neurotransmitters**), particularly **dopamine** and **norepinephrine**. These substances allow our *billions* of brain cells to communicate, one to another, creating neural pathways along which information and instructions travel. **To say that "we're wired differently," refers to these information-laden neural pathways. This expression is almost literal!**

Depending on which regions of the brain are low in dopamine and/or norepinephrine, the ADHD mind races, working extra hard to try to accomplish the tasks associated with those regions.

Stimulant medications, the most common type of ADHD medication, increase the brain's access to these neurotransmitters, bolstering the flow of information from cell to cell along the neural pathways.

As counterintuitive as it seems, ADHD stimulant meds don't speed up an ADHDer. Instead, with more neurotransmitters on hand, the brain's regions interact more easily, easing the struggle to communicate with each other.

All of which is to say, ADHD is real, and whatever you do to increase your wellness, will ultimately help your ADHD. The brain is part of the physical body!

Many of the entries in Part IV are intended to help you in one way or another.

Mind, body, and spirit are connected, so, hopefully, reading this book should be good for your general health!

Find an ADHD Coach

I've never had an ADHD coach per se, but for about a year around the time I was diagnosed, I worked with a therapist *as an ADHD coach*. (I've also had an ADHD buddy.)

If you can possibly get it together, have the means, etc., I believe that you could only benefit from having a coach. (I consider therapy or coaching not a sign of weakness, but a privileged advantage.) **Maybe you can find an inexpensive option; set aside a lump of money for a limited series of sessions; do less costly group coaching; or have a single session to get you headed in the right direction.**

Below are half a dozen sites you can check out to learn a lot more about what coaching can do and some coaches who do it.

- *ADDCA, Accredited ADHD & Life Coach Training Program*

    Under *Find a Coach* on ADDCA's homepage, you will see a couple of featured coaches. From there, go to the bottom of that page, and under *Find Coaches By*, click on *Women*, or *Adult* or whatever else you're particularly interested in to see a long list of coaches who specialize in that area.

- **Expert ADHD Coaching**

    This place has about 25 coaches on staff, including its founder, Shanna Pearson. You can read all their bios in the drop-down menu under *Our Expert ADHD Team* on the site's homepage. You can also get a free initial consult by filling out a form under *Contact Us* on the homepage.

- **CADDAC, Center for ADHD Awareness, Canada**

    To find a list of ADHD group coaches, click on *Programs & Events* on CADDAC's homepage and then *Group Coaching Programs*. Remember, with virtual coaching, you don't have to be in the same country as your coach or the other participants! The CADDAC site also has a great deal of information and resources for people with ADHD of all ages.

- **iACTcenter, The International ADHD Coach Training Center**

    This site was founded by ADHD coach and author, Laurie Dupar. Under *Hire a Coach*, you can check out a list of ADHD coaches, their bios, and how they work with people. Dupar no longer coaches one on one, but she does offer a *Pick My Brain* phone call ($135) during which you can ask her anything.

- **Hallowell ADHD Centers**

    The Centers' founder, Dr. Edward ("Ned") Hallowell, is a pioneer in the field of ADHD, has ADHD himself, appears to be very friendly, and is a great champion of all ADHDers. He's the author or co-author of numerous books, including *Driven to Distraction*, and is arguably the most well-known and knowledgeable speaker on ADHD in the western world. Hallowell has a number of centers across the U.S., including those in New York City, the Boston area, California's Bay Area, and Seattle. And, with the advent of telehealth, you can connect with the centers from anywhere in the world.

Under *Services* on the main page of his site, you can click on *Coaching* and find and fill out a short form to ask for a free (no pressure) *New Patient Consult* with one of the organization's clinicians (whose bios you can read on the site).

- **Terry Maitland, MSW,** is a psychotherapist, well-respected ADHD expert, coach, and author of the wonderful book, *Queen of Distraction*. Check out her site for a list of ways she can help you, information on membership in her *Queens of Distraction* group, and many links to resources for women with ADHD. Her blog is also up to date and has many great, personal posts about ADHD. To see how Terry works with people one on one, click on *ADHD Consulting* on her site's homepage.

- **Diane O'Reilly, Your Real ADHD Life Coach**

  This is the site of ADHD coach Diane O'Reilly. I don't know her, but I love the encouraging and uplifting material she presents about women with ADHD on her homepage. To book an initial call, click the button that says *Book a Call* on the top right of her site.

- *Getting Clear Coaching with ADHD Coach, Linda Anderson, MA, MCC*

    Linda is an experienced ADHD coach. She's a member, former president, and board member of the Attention Deficit Disorder Association (ADDA). Her site, *Getting Clear*, has a lot of helpful information on ADHD. On its homepage alone, there are lists of how you could benefit from having a coach; what you could accomplish with a coach; and what she can offer you as a coach. For a free, no pressure intro talk, contact Linda in the short form under *Contact* on her homepage.

One last idea: Almost all the websites and organizations mentioned in the entry *Find a Therapist, Part III*, have information that could guide you to finding a coach.

Find an ADHD Buddy

I love women with ADHD. I feel so at home with them, so accepted. At ease. Free to be myself.

Typically, an ADHD buddy is someone you meet up with to help you stay accountable for things you're doing. I've had a couple over the years and found it so useful and encouraging. I highly recommend you giving it a try.

It's the same magic that's at the heart of all *12-Step Programs*: **Something miraculous is created when two people come together over a shared experience.**

There are so many ways to find women with ADHD online now and hopefully you can find some who live near you, too. I've connected with a bunch of women I've encountered on Instagram and who have written to me about my first book. I've interviewed women with ADHD to get their stories to tell here. I've had women with ADHD therapists (two), and I happen to know a lot of women with ADHD.

You can almost always recognize them: They're often enthusiastic, kind, and full of ideas but not always speedy (like I am). Sometimes they're poised and dreamy like two friends of mine. Often, they have a big heart. They can be adventurous, creative, empathetic, curious, resourceful, and willing to jump on board with you for whatever it is.

I hope you find a buddy.

Get Connected

*"My best friend and I met in California where we both grew up a couple blocks from each other, and when I moved away 3-ish years ago, we wanted to find a way to stay connected that would kind of work as a reminder for each other that we were still alive. So we found a dominoes app that allows us to just play a domino when we have the time. I think this app was instrumental in keeping us really connected. Especially now that I know I am ADHD, because the notification that she had played a domino at least daily reminded me she was still there, and **I have a really hard time remembering to stay in contact with people that are not frequently around me.** So having a game that we played back and forth constantly was an easy and noninvasive reminder."*

—Jessica from Oregon

One of my biggest struggles is getting myself out there connecting with people. Yet nothing buoys me up to keep on keeping on more than talking, meeting with, or even just texting someone. **Connecting reminds me that I'm part of something bigger than myself and not alone.**

A July 28, 2010, article in *Scientific American* by Katherine Harmon, entitled *Social Ties Boost Survival by 50 Percent,* reported that **social connections with others—family, friends, work buddies—is as good for health as giving up a 15-cigarette-a-day habit!** These results were based on a review of 148 different studies that covered more than 300,000 people of all ages.

ADHDer Dr. Ned (Edward) Hallowell, likely the most well-known ADHD expert, psychiatrist, and author, thinks that getting connected is one of most beneficial things any ADHDer can do. And, this is absolutely true for me!

Aside from having an ADHD buddy, therapist, or coach, **below are different ways you can get yourself out there and connect with the world.** It always makes me feel better when I do.

- **Find Your Third Place.**

    The third place refers to someplace you can go to regularly that's not work or home, but a third place. For me, it's easy: I'm a café lover. I always find a café I can drop into and shoot the breeze with a bunch of friends and acquaintances. I see them day in and day out. I know them and they know me. I love that: being held in the minds of a group of people. I think of them when I'm not there and imagine good things happening for them (even just the acquaintances).

- **Really Listen and Take in What People are Saying.**

    We're so busy so much of the time. Often, we're bubbling over with a strong need to say what we want to say, which distracts us from really listening to other people. Some psychology professionals consider giving your attention to another to be a genuine act of love. I think of it that way. Needing to be heard and acknowledged is a basic human need and works both ways: you talking and you listening. Practice being present and listening, really listening, to what the other guy is saying.

- **Deepen Your Small Talk with an Acquaintance if it Seems Safe.**

    Small talk is fun, it's good, and I love it. But I also keep an eye out for an opening when I might reveal something deeper about myself or experience. It's liberating for others to hear what another person is tackling. Often, this level of realness uplifts the other person. Western society expects us to put on a happy face. But people need to acknowledge emotionally challenging issues. Sharing a problem with a safe friend, or even a new friend, can change my head in a few minutes. I can go from feeling isolated and lost, to empowered and renewed, after talking about a difficult issue. I don't mean talking about being a victim or complaining negatively about your bad life. That doesn't help me. But having someone share their feelings about the issues they're working through—or me mine—can buoy me and fortify me emotionally.

- **If You Remotely Qualify for any *12-Step Program*, try some meetings.**

    Man, 12-Step programs can be a hard sell. But if you remotely qualify for any of them—do yourself a favor and check out some meetings. You don't have to say a word to anyone if you don't want to. There are no bosses or rules. If you're not having some kind of addiction issue, but grew up with dysfunction or live or work with it, you might try *Al-anon*. All meetings are different—so check out a few before deciding if they're good for you or not. There are thousands online. If you feel self-conscious going, pretend you're a reporter covering the issue!

- **Seek Out a *Meetup* Group on Something You Love.**

    Go to Meetup.com and see if there are any groups on subjects you like or want to know more about. It's so much fun to have fun ... or share interests with others.

- **Consider a Church.**

    I know people who don't have a particular belief in a God but go to church for the community. I'm aware that organized religion has turned a lot of people off in the past, including me. Still, I'm now absolutely sure that there are dogma-free churches with great communities. Maybe you can find one.

- **Pick up the Phone and Make That Call.**

    Man, do I have a hard time calling people. I don't know why. I'm shyish I guess. I'm also often awkward on the phone. Or afraid someone is going to demand something of me that I don't want to give. Or, maybe I'm afraid I can't handle the other person's pain. I don't know. But I'm working on it. After I call my older aunt, I feel so good!

Work on Acceptance and Allowing

I just had dinner with some old friends who were visiting from California. They're the sweetest couple. The wife, I'll call her Emily, is an artist who loves life: She said she can't wait to get to sleep at night so she can wake up the next morning and start doing things again. She doesn't seem to have any depression, definitely doesn't have ADHD, has had money all her adult life, and, I've just found out, has recently moved into a house that is my true dream home.

So, I'm feeling a painful envy now that tells me that I'll never be able to create the beauty she has in her environment: that I just don't have it in me.

Clearly, she doesn't struggle with feeling overwhelmed. Or deciding priorities. Or depression. Or ultra sensitivity.

So, I'm sitting here having to work on my acceptance of who and what I am. Again. I know I can do it: I've done it lots of times before.

Yup: Some people look like they've really got it made. And maybe they do. I don't know how it all works. But I do know that **comparing myself to someone else is never-ending and**

pointless. There's always someone worse off and someone better off. Where will comparing get me?

Until I accept any hard thing I encounter, I know I won't be able to embrace any healing/helping moves.

Accepting the fact that you've got difficulties with ADHD is one of the first steps to being able to move forward. **But, how to do it?**

I'm going to start right now, in this situation I'm in, by having compassion for myself for going through this pain. I know I'm not alone in feeling "less than," like I do right this minute.

I'm letting myself feel it—and taking a deep breath.

Knowing that I'm not the only person to feel this kind of pain helps.

I don't know why some people are homeless or starving while others live at the center of an abundant life, seemingly overflowing with happiness, love, kids, creativity, health, money, and sunshine. And, I know I'll never have these answers.

Already, I'm feeling a bit better. A bit more accepting. There's so much I can't know. But I do know that I can only work with what I am, what's in my own head and on my plate.

I see myself right now as a hurting child and my heart goes out to myself! **I want to accept all of myself. I know that I need to love myself because if I'm not going to be on my own side, be loyal to myself, and want myself, then who will?**

I say the Serenity Prayer because it cuts through so much.

God, grant me the serenity (and power) to accept the things I cannot change,
The courage (and power) to change the things I can,
And the wisdom (and power) to know the difference.

I breathe deeply and feel a little better.

Watch Your Hormones

"Women suffer more than men in the roller coaster of ADHD symptoms because of our monthly hormone cycles and how they impact the availability of neurotransmitters and chemicals in our brains.

Anyway, the sage wisdom coming out of the ADHD community is to pay close attention and track your monthly cycle and to plan your life carefully around it. This doesn't mean only when you bleed, what this means is to learn to understand how our energy levels and thought processes are impacted throughout the month.

This is a HUGE thing I am trying to learn and study, as I have two daughters who will soon join my ranks in this monthly rollercoaster, and I want to pass on wisdom not shame about how this will really feel and look."

—Anastasia, wife and working mom

Before deciding on the title for my first book, *Help for Women with ADHD: My Simple Strategies for Conquering Chaos*, the working title I used was *Is it PMS, Menopause, or Verifiable ADHD?: My Simple Strategies for Conquering Chaos*.

I'd been calling it that because I so clearly saw that a lot of women who didn't have ADHD seemed like they did when they were in the thick of PMS and perimenopause. You know, **complaining that they couldn't think, felt overwhelmed, got easily emotionally triggered, felt anxious or depressed, all that.**

But what I hadn't considered back then was how those changes also affected women who actually have ADHD!

Like Anastasia (above) says, PMS can make a woman's challenging ADHD traits worse at certain times. As can perimenopause and menopause.

The hormonal piece of the puzzle for women with ADHD isn't widely considered yet, but some wise women and doctors out there understand how it likely works.

Not that it's rocket science: If you've had PMS, menopause, or perimenopause, you have likely felt the ride hormones can take you on.

Throughout a woman's 28-day menstrual cycle, estrogen and progesterone wax and wane.

For the first two weeks, beginning with Day 1 of your period, estrogen starts building up. And estrogen enhances the action of at least two of our "feel good" brain chemicals (aka neurotransmitters)—serotonin and dopamine.

Meanwhile, though, in the second two weeks of the menstrual cycle, progesterone builds up, muting estrogen's enhancing effects.

In perimenopause, the hormonal dance isn't regular at all, but up and down and all over the place.

And after menopause, there's a general lessening of estrogen.

As always, awareness is a first step toward working on a problem. If you're able to chart your monthly ups and downs over several months, you may see behavioral patterns.

From there, you may use various strategies for handling the times when you know you're going to need more help: Maybe you can get harder things done before your PMS hits, exercise more, or ask someone for help.

Some women end up taking oral contraceptives to regulate hormonal fluctuations.

Others take a bit more of their ADHD medication on the tough days of the month.

Others have found fish oil to be helpful as well as estrogen-like supplements such as Remifemin, which is made from the black cohosh plant. There's also always the possibility of taking bio-identical hormone replacement therapy in perimenopause or after menopause (If you decide to take bio-identical hormones, it's essential that you begin taking them within a year of the start of menopause for them to be effective.)

You're going to have to be your own advocate and researcher to find help with this. Connect with other women and see what wisdom and guidance they may share. (You might want to search for articles or recorded talks with Dr. Jeanette Wasserstein, a neuropsychologist who is one of the few voices out there sharing on this subject.)

Get Educated About ADHD

"Well, for the past two decades, since my 20s, I have been looking for ways to improve myself. Make myself better, more productive, more focused, more organized, less overwhelmed, more patient, more fit, more of just about everything! In looking back, especially over the last decade, **I am aghast that before now not one thing I read, or one professional I sought help from ever led me down the path of determining whether I have ADHD.** *Since then, I have immersed myself in articles, books, and podcasts that talk of this very real problem, and yet I see a huge glaring gap that still exists in the world of information that doesn't connect the dots for us ADHDers."*

—Anastasia, wife and working mom

There's so much ignorance out there about ADHD and other neurodivergent, "invisible" differences. Even a lot of people who think they know about ADHD, don't have a clue (sorry).

Because I've learned a lot about the subject, I've become pretty good at enlightening people I meet who say ridiculous, shaming things about ADHD, or simply don't know one true thing about it.

Often, when I've been able to say something informative, people who'd previously believed ADHD was the same as a Type A personality or some other ignorant thing, get a look of understanding in their eyes.

But because there are so many parts to the condition, it's difficult to get your thoughts together to convey what it is when you're out somewhere and run into the ignorance problem.

That's why **I think it's a good idea to have a few sentences ready to offer up in situations when people belittle ADHD.** I've found that doing that really changes the direction of the conversation. Not only that, but it builds self-esteem to set the record straight and stand up for ourselves and others.

Below are a few ideas you might incorporate into what you figure out to say to people you encounter who don't know anything about ADHD, or worse, say it doesn't exist.

- "One of the basic differences about someone with ADHD is that we have a wide-open focus that takes in ten times more of everything than the average person. Think what a kid would be like in a toy store. The average neurotypical person, on the other hand, naturally grays out most of their surroundings except what they're focused on. This seeing so much all around us all the time is very distracting for ADHDers because not only are we aware of so much, but our minds feel they have to do something about all that we see."
- "Some people describe ADHD as having a mind that has many radio stations on at the same time."
- "Although there's no single test for ADHD like there is for heart disease or diabetes, science considers ADHD a

biology-based condition that has to do with the way our brain cells communicate with each other. This is what we mean when we ADHDers say that we're wired differently. This different wiring gives people with ADHD different focusing abilities that play out in a range of different traits."
- "The different wiring of the ADHD brain is responsible for both challenges and tremendous assets, including high levels of creativity and innovative, out-of-the-box thinking."
- "There's a lot to ADHD that makes it hard to explain quickly but one thing to remember is that ADHD is a spectrum condition, which means some ADHDers have some traits and not others. By the same token, all humans experience all the traits ADHDers do, just not as strongly as those who really have ADHD."

So there!

Connect with a Greater Good Beyond Yourself

On your death bed, what will you want to remember about how you spent your time on Earth?

I was diagnosed with ADHD as an adult about 20 years ago.

I'm overwhelmingly grateful I was diagnosed. That awareness prompted me to learn about ADHD, find help, and discover various ways to harness its hard parts and recognize its good parts.

For me, one of the greatest things that learning about ADHD has given me has been learning to identify priorities.

I never used to think about priorities. Now, I usually figure out *what I need or want to do the most* on any given day. This helps me avoid being tossed around from one impulse to another like a ping pong ball.

And priorities don't end with day-to-day priority setting. Not by a long shot. They work on a higher, lifelong level.

I think a person's ultimate priority is akin to her personal philosophy: What do you want to live for, going into the future, that will give your life meaning?

I think I might have never pinned this down if I hadn't gotten help for my ADHD. I might have been too busy catching up and putting out fires to establish a life philosophy.

What do *you* want to live for?

- Maybe it's self realization—a dedication to aligning with creative consciousness or God.
- Maybe it's giving love to a child.
- Maybe it's promoting an environmentally-sound vision of life on earth.
- Maybe it's giving to others in particular ways.
- Maybe it's developing a talent or art.
- Maybe it's a commitment to your own recovery and healing, yours and others'.
- Maybe it's helping your one neighbor.
- Maybe it's spending your life working on forgiveness and appreciation, as a spiritual practice.

Usually, it involves doing something that connects you to a greater good beyond yourself.

Having an overarching purpose and staying faithful to it going forward ensures that all your lost projects and unkempt yards will fade away in time.

In the end, it won't be how good you looked or what a high achiever you were. It will always be about something or someone you stood for, no matter the circumstances.

Everything in this book has helped me get to this point of knowing my priorities and excavating the treasure of existence: recognizing what I love enough to live for.

Safeguard Your Feelings

"*I didn't really know what I liked or didn't like,*" said a woman I spoke to who has ADHD. She'd been raised with a demanding mother who knew nothing about ADHD. Having always tried to please her as a kid, she grew into a woman who wasn't sure where she stood on a number of issues. It wasn't until she got into her first serious relationship that she began to realize that the chronic criticism she grew up with had stunted her development.

This is a sad story a lot of us can relate to. It makes me angry, so I want to make sure you know that I firmly believe that ***absolutely no one can tell you what you should like or not like.***

No one can tell you what you should or shouldn't be feeling, either. Sad, mad, glad, or happy, your feelings aren't up for debate or criticism.

Feelings aren't good or bad or facts to be debated. What I like and don't like is always okay and only my business.

It's totally inappropriate in every situation for someone to judge another person's preferences or feelings.

Stick with people who honor your feelings, whatever they are.

Plenty of neurodivergent women have lost their voice from years of feeling like they didn't fit in.

It is always enough and an exactly healthy response to simply like something. You do not have to justify to anyone why you like anything.

If this sounds like you, you might love the wisdom in Melody Beattie's classic *The Language of Letting Go: Daily Meditations for Codependents*. (It's listed in the *Resources* section at the end of this book.)

Play

"I get 10 new hobbies a month, some work, most don't, but I love exploring. I am so hands-on trying to create, make something, and use my hands. I can usually fix something in a different way than a 'normal' person would."

—Selina Danielle, U.K.

I follow this cute woman with ADHD on Instagram who reminds me of Selina.

She's in her early 30s and just talks about what's going on with her. She's funny and has a very expressive face. She has a supportive, positive attitude about having ADHD.

Anyway, as I was watching her strumming a ukulele one day, it hit me how important playing is for adults. You don't hear about playing much in our society. But **many health professionals promote adult play as a healthy way to unwind, relax, soothe the brain, feed creativity, and more.**

It's interesting that many dot-com and other top companies with big campuses (offices) promote employee play by offering various options like ping pong tables, yoga classes, and recess times. The leadership at these billion-dollar companies knows that adult play ultimately increases the company's bottom line and capacity for innovation.

For women with ADHD, playing is especially beneficial! Play gives us a free pass to explore all the interesting activities that constantly flit through our wide-open awareness—in an unstructured way.

The idea with play is that you're not attempting to accomplish anything, you're just playing around.

The point of play is just to play. You don't have to be good at the activity.

Playing can be anything that's fun or interesting to you: making stuff, exploring connections, checking on something, cooking, beading, drawing, playing an instrument, singing, dancing, gardening, learning a new piece of software, gaming, sewing, knitting, crocheting, decorating, painting, examining something new, working with clay, going to a park and taking a slide or a swing. Flying a kite or building an altar in a corner somewhere. Climbing a tree or sitting under one. Rigging up a tent in the living room. Coloring.

Playing gives you permission to pursue any interest in a playful way *without having to produce anything from the effort*. You don't try to succeed at anything when playing: You don't have to finish playing or win anything. If you did, it wouldn't be playing!

Play is so freeing, especially for people like us who have so many interests.

Have a creative life. Give yourself playtimes and live into the creative chaos! Indulge in your natural inclination to explore things.

So: I play the guitar. Not well, but well enough to get pleasure from it. I make jewelry, too. I sew, knit, and crochet some. The other day I made a new cover for a daily reader book I love. It came out almost perfectly, but not quite: I didn't know to leave more room for the spine! I also recently made a felt liner for a tote bag. I glued it to the inside of the bag.

Before I finally settled on journalism, editing and writing, I was employed as a restaurant server, a cook, an actress, a guitar teacher, a bench jeweler, a director of development for an amazing environmental non-profit, and the creative director for a company, run by a crazed woman, that produced fruit-flavored perfume for kids!

You?

Grieve

"At this point, it became apparent that both my childhood and adult behavior could be explained by hyperactive ADHD, combined with emotional dysregulation, and the most effective form of treatment was to take prescribed medication.

I felt like my world had blown up in front of my eyes and I couldn't stop crying. I had been cheated. All the missed opportunities to develop my career; to be known as an expert in a bespoke profession came swarming back into my head and I was devasted. Why now? Why had it taken 32 years to get here?"

—Sara, 36, U.K.

After being misdiagnosed repeatedly and getting the runaround for several years in the U.K. health system, our Sara, above, finally got a diagnosis of ADHD.

Like so many other women—many of whom weren't diagnosed until their 30s, 40s, 50s, 60s, 70s or 80s—Sara was both angry and grief-stricken at first. After adjusting to ADHD meds, which work wonderfully for her, and seeing a therapist, Sara had been at the same job for three years when I talked with her and was doing really well.

Women have a range of initial reactions to the knowledge that they have ADHD: One of them is grief.

Grief is a deep sadness people feel when they come face to face with a loss: the break-up of a marriage or friendship; the death of a loved one; the loss of a job; environmental degradation; a health diagnosis.

Some people can't handle their grief and repress it and rush over it into some kind of action. But repressed emotions usually end up coming out sideways: You might become bitter about life, mean to others, depressed, closed off, or totally shut down.

Ultimately, most of us have to grieve our losses, whatever they are, in order to move on.

It's only through acceptance that we can make peace with reality and start working to make things better from *where and who we are and what we have.*

If you are newly diagnosed, do you feel sad about it? I get it. It's natural. I hope you can let yourself grieve.

There's no one way to sit with painful feelings. Sharing them with other safe people helps me enormously. Sharing truthfully about some hard thing I'm going through can help my sadness start to shift and allow me to begin to glimpse a way forward.

When you're able to be vulnerable and honest with others, you often find that you're not alone in your grief: that the other person is carrying some themselves. And then you feel for them and that opens your heart.

And in your opened heart all kinds of feelings rush out: joy to have a bond with another; happiness that you've helped someone else; a sense of awe that life is all that life is; and much, much more.

That's the theory. I've experienced it myself.

Know that Every Little Bit Adds Up

If we could only have the patience to understand, grasp, and embody this core truth about living, learning, growing, and life: Every little bit counts. If we could, we'd know that even **if we can only work on our ADHD challenges a little right now, we're still going in the right direction!**

I've watched my husband polish his language skills by reading Italian newspapers and books, little by little, every day for the 30 years I've known him. He's as fluent as our Italian nieces and nephew.

I want to be like that. My tendency is to think things have to be done all at once, hard!

It's January 2019, and I've been working on writing this book and giving it a good form for a couple months. It feels like a very big and unwieldy task.

But I want to work the every-little-bit-adds-up strategy because I've seen that you can build something big, a little bit at a time!

So, I'm trying to remember that as I try (pray) to stay with this project, day in and day out, a little bit at a time.

Whatever you're doing to change for the better adds up.

Humans never stop growing and changing, so the question is not whether you're going to grow, but whether you want to grow toward the good (the Light), or not.

One way to grow yourself better (healthier, happier) is to understand that every little bit counts and adds up. **Nothing good is lost.**

Dismantle Shame

'I started to pay attention to my personal narrative and realized that most of the things I let pile up were triggering a negative personal belief and it was causing me to shut down and walk away from the tasks. **I would hear myself immediately say in my mind things like, "I never can finish what I start," "I am too stupid to do this task," "I suck so why even try?" "You aren't smart enough for this."**

—Anastasia, wife and working mom

"No shame in being an addict," this gorgeous guy used to regularly, nicely, yell out/interject when everybody would be clapping about something at a 12-Step meeting I went to 20 years ago.

I loved him for that. I loved the **courageous vulnerability** in his declarations.

Shame is this big, deep, heavy thing most humans get sometimes after having done something we judge to be wrong.

Sometimes we feel ashamed because we actually have committed a wrong: said something mean, neglected someone in need, lied to cover our asses. In those cases, the shame cues us into amending our actions or apologizing for them.

But, way too often, we feel ashamed about just being ourselves: *We feel that we're not good enough in some way. In any way. In many ways.*

Baseless shame is a dark thing that the mindfulness teacher, author, and therapist Tara Brach calls a "trance of unworthiness."

And plenty of women with ADHD have even more of this mistaken and debilitating shame than the average person.

It starts when growing up without the tools you need to bridge the gap between your fluid mind and society's expected and codified way of doing things.

Lots of us have spent a lot of time being criticized for not doing this or that exactly like others.

Why this happens isn't surprising when you consider that societies and cultures develop dominant, conventional standards of behavior. And society's worst voice criticizes those who don't fit! And so it starts: this misperceived sense of self.

This backlog of low self-esteem is a heavy load to carry.

I love this woman, Sari Solden, a well-known author, ADHD expert, and therapist, for being a fierce advocate of the fact that our self worth is inherent and distinctly separate from our brain-based differences.

I'm with her!

We need to shore up our self-esteem so we're clear about the fact that—separate from our ADHD—we're whole people unquestionably worthy of giving and receiving love.

Which is why I celebrate and strive to normalize neurodiverse ways of being human.

Two things I know about dismantling shame is that it's an ongoing effort (like bailing out a leaky boat) and that being brave enough to share your vulnerable feelings with safe people starts you on the road to recovery.

It's our job to combat the remnants of the ignorance that has surrounded all mental and emotional health issues for centuries. Brain-based conditions are just as real as the ones we consider body-based and there's no shame in them, just as there's no shame attached to people with cancer or diabetes.

Take that inner road. Dismantle your shame. Fly your flag!

Strive for Simplicity

ADHDers have a strong attraction to the here and now. That's why whatever is in front of me, in the present moment, gets an oversized portion of my attention and energy.

Objects snag my attention and make me feel like I have to do something about them. My energy gets all congested when I have too many things.

Simplicity for me is all about avoiding having my focus caught by objects that are out of place, that I haven't used for ages, or are all disorganized. Plenty of people have no problem at all with this, but I do.

When I can simplify and declutter various areas of my physical surroundings, I'm left feeling free of that nagging sense of being overwhelmed.

Which is why I keep things as spare as possible in my house.

I'm currently, once again, purging clothing from my closet. I have some beautiful clothing, but I wear basically a handful of items. So, I've just taken a bunch of clothes I cannot bear to give away and put them in another closet where I don't have to see them. I've also just managed to take a big bag of clothes to our local thrift shop.

Having fewer things in my closet makes it much easier to choose what I'm going to wear.

With fewer options, I don't become confused by all the clothing I'd love to wear but don't wear for one reason or another: items that may need mending, or altering, washing, or are wrinkled.

Having fewer items in my closet also helps me see good options to wear that I otherwise wouldn't notice when the closet is packed.

Having fewer clothes in my closet is like being on vacation and having only a limited number of things to wear. I always love that.

The clutter problem is tough across the board. For me, it's a background anxiety that I have to take care of a bunch of things: restring my boots, toss out bad leftovers in the refrigerator, get rid of storage container lids, hem a dress, clean my car. Just writing this makes me anxious. (I know all these things are inconsequential in the scheme of things, but the effect they have on me is not inconsequential, so I have to deal with it.)

Whenever I clean the refrigerator, I feel so much better, it motivates me to cook and make a good meal.

This goes on and on. There are tons of great people out there helping women with ADHD (and others) learn how to keep things spare.

It feels like I'll never get there, and maybe I won't. But every inroad I make in simplifying the physical objects I have by analyzing what I need and getting rid of the rest helps me feel more free.

You get it, right?

The Value of Failure

Have you ever come across the concept that **the road to success is lined with failure?**

All the big "productivity" gurus talk about it. And now **an institute at Columbia University**—*Education for Persistence and Innovation Center (EPIC)*—**is studying how successful people bounce back from failure!**

In a 2016 study, the director of the institute (Dr. Xiaodong Lin) found that sharing stories with students about the failures of celebrities increased their ability to tackle their own failures.

According to Dr. Lin, if you only impart academic knowledge to students, but don't teach them how to keep going after failing, their academic achievements won't be enough.

I'm really thrilled to know about this institute.

Among the secrets to benefiting from a failure is that failure contains information that helps you make a smarter attempt next time.

Not only that, but experts believe that the more failed attempts you make at something, the better the chances that you will ultimately succeed.

Sadly, though, for a lot of us, failing at something is the end of the particular thing we were attempting. Failure often flattens sensitive people making us feel defeated and causing us to give up.

But the name of the game (of life) is to know that failure is part of the process of succeeding at what you are trying to do—and getting back up on that horse (as the saying goes) is the wise move!

The great writer and speaker **Brené Brown's work mirrors these ideas**. She's an academic who's spent decades studying vulnerability and shame. One of her main prescriptions is that a person is unlikely to achieve anything worthwhile, or real, unless they are courageous enough *to be willing to fail.*

I was an actress in my 20s and looking back, I saw that a lot of the people who got jobs were not more talented than others. It was that they just kept auditioning consistently, day in and day out.

Sometimes the resilience is instinctive, but often it arises from studying what experts have to say about the value of failure. Which is what we're doing here.

Spirit Power/Higher Flower

Do you have a higher flower—I mean, a higher power?

Are you a believer?

By that, I mean do you believe in **a power greater than yourself?** In a field of **creative intelligence? The Universe? In a source of good? In a "God" of your own understanding?**

If you're lucky enough to be open to prayer, capitalize on it and get real about spending some quiet time doing it.

Prayer helps me. Really helps me. The remarkable thing is that you can pray even though you don't know exactly what or who you're praying to!

Mostly my prayers are filled with gratitude for all the good in my life or pleas to help me and help other people I know or love. Almost always, a while after I've prayed, I'll suddenly realize that my problem issues have shifted for me—in a good way.

It doesn't hurt to remember that plenty of people think that humans are spiritual beings having a physical experience. And that the majority of people on Earth believe in some kind of a Higher Power/God.

I love how Elizabeth Gilbert, in her beautiful memoir *Eat, Pray, Love*, realized for herself that "God" was "in her, as her."

In her, as her.

Build Your Toolbox and Leave the Rest

Even though I've written that you'd do well if you did a whole bunch of things to tackle your difficult ADHD traits, I'm going to contradict myself here.

Each of us is different and resonates with different things. We're unique in ways we can't even see, so don't feel like there's something wrong with you if you have no interest in various suggestions in this book.

Like what you like, and don't worry about the other stuff: Take what you want and leave the rest, reader.

There's no way everything fits everybody!

Not only that, but if you just can't get into working on yourself in any which way, just forget about it! You're okay, no matter what!

PART IV

Strategies, Tips, Hacks, and Helpful Things You Can Apply to Your Life

The entries here contain tips, tools, strategies, and suggestions that help me manage the whirling chaos of the world.

They're lightly subdivided into "Organization," "Time Management," "Self Knowledge," "Self-care," "Feelings," and "Relationships."

PART IV A

Organization, Planning, and Memory

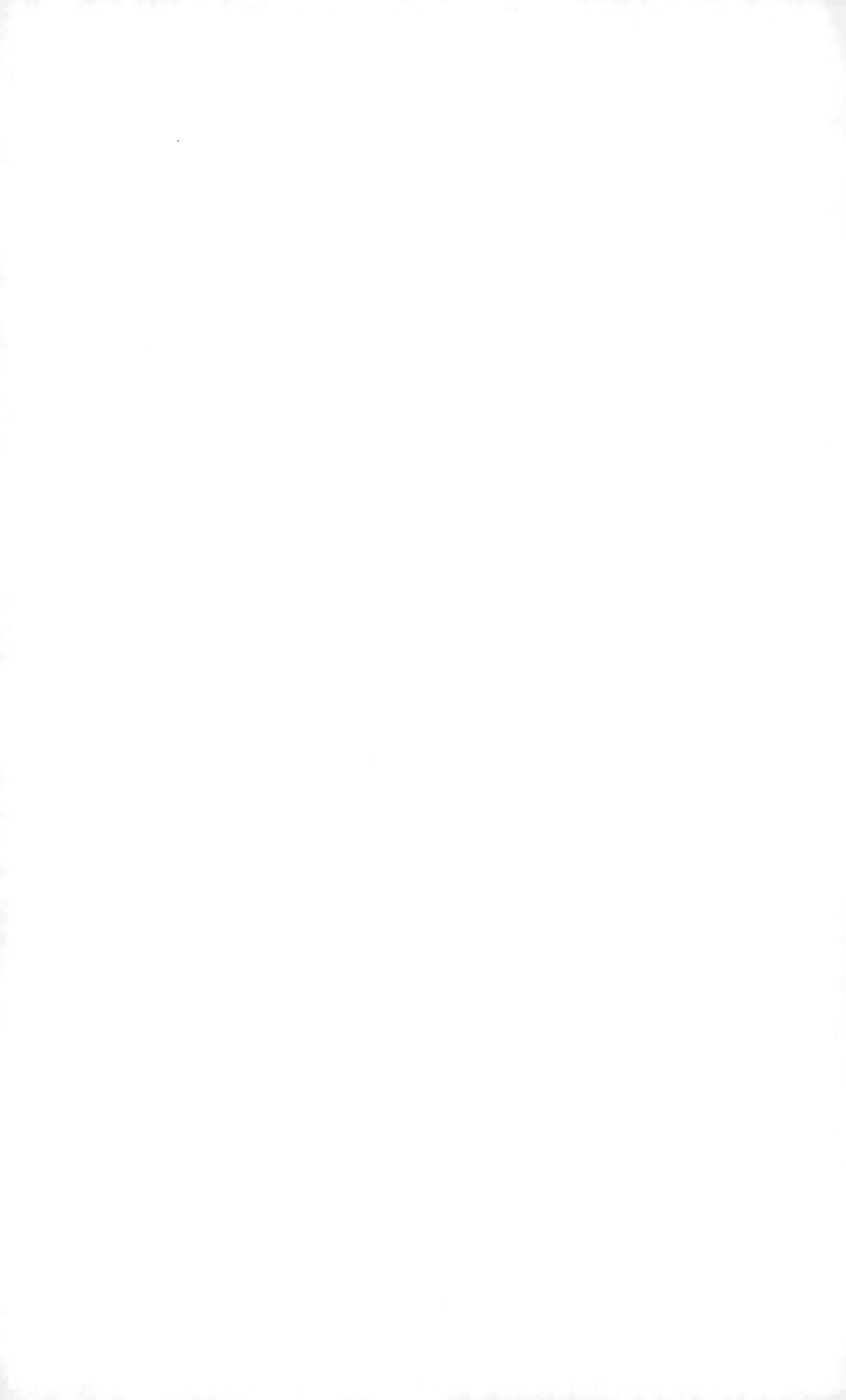

Landing Pad

I've been getting worse at hanging on to my phone in my house lately. So I've just re-implemented my landing pad strategy, **designating three new homes for my (f*cking/fantastic) phone.**

I use these spots for other items that I also want to remember to take with me when I go out.

I have a special spot downstairs, one upstairs, and one in my bag.

So, applying this to my phone, here's how I'm doing it: Every single time I move my phone, **I have to put it back in one of the three landing/launching pads:** Upstairs, it's a stool/small table-like thing in the hallway. Downstairs, it's a small countertop area in the kitchen where I keep a jar of pens, my keys, and sunglasses, too.

And the last location is a bag I now carry. It's a small shoulder strap bag that I often carry inside another bag—a big tote. And the phone goes in the small bag—not just anywhere in the tote.

So, that's it. If I lose the phone, it should be in one of those three places.

I just keep putting the phone in these designated spots. And if I don't do it, and can't find the phone, when I do find it, I put it back in one of the places for at least a few minutes.

It's working!

Use External Cues

*"One thing I got from a friend with ADHD: **I got a whiteboard. It's drilled into my bedroom wall, which is my office now: a big white board.***

And she had me divide it into Today, This Week, and Someday.

Which has been pretty helpful, and I try to use two different color pens: one for work stuff, and one for home life and personal stuff. And it's pretty good. Although I can definitely walk right by it sometimes! **But it's right there, so if I have a thought, I can write it down and it's not lost in some drawer.** *So that's been helpful.*

I do think a real calendar helps, but you have to keep it in one place. And Post-it notes… I keep them around me all the time and put them on my laptop."

—Sarah, writer, a child psychologist, and mother of two in the Bay Area

I'd love to have a room with whiteboards for walls!

I find external cues—by which I mean things you can write, draw, or otherwise construct and physically hang up around you—so useful!

The reason why external cues, like white boards, are especially useful for people with ADHD has to do with the idea that ADHD traits result from a weakness in a group of internal cueing abilities known as executive functions.

These cueing functions operate almost automatically beneath the conscious mind. They include the ability to mentally juggle and remember—*over a span of time in the back of the mind*—all the parts of a task we're undertaking so we can act on the many components needed to complete it. They also include various cognitive processes that allow us to regulate our attention; to track our progress on an effort; to sort and organize thoughts; to envision a finished project, and to regulate strong emotions, like frustration, so as to maintain focus on a task at hand.

So, given that these internal cues are less than robust in many people with ADHD, it makes perfect sense for us to shore up their functioning with external, physical cues—right where they can see them!

Like big **whiteboards, Post-it notes, signs, collages, vision boards** or any other physical representation that reminds you of what you want to keep on your mind. (Be creative!)

Analog clocks are also a helpful type of external cue for time myopia—seeing the hands helps. Get a few and put them all over the place.

Know, too, that deficits in our executive functioning have nothing to do with how intelligent we may be: We just need some support keeping that intelligence on tract and headed in a chosen direction.

Boom!

Desk Notebook (Info Capture System)

I couldn't handle myself and all the world requires if I didn't have a central place where I can capture information for safe keeping. **I can't just jot something down on a scrap of paper thinking I'll remember where it is.**

My indispensable, main, go-to tool is what I call my *desk notebook*.

Although it's just a simple notebook, two things magically transform my *desk notebook* into a sophisticated (i.e., highly functional) information storage system.

First is that I use it exclusively to jot everything down.

And second is that I look through the notebook at least once a day.

I recommend against buying a fancy one—although I do love Moleskins. But whichever one you buy, you want one you feel free to be sloppy in! I like medium-sized notebooks, which are around 5-inch by 8-inch, depending on the brand. (Just FYI, this size is considerably smaller than a standard 8 ½-inch by 11-inch sheet of paper.)

As soon as I start a new notebook (because I've filled up an old one), I use a large marker (either on the cover itself or on a piece of masking tape on the cover) and write *desk notebook* and the date.

And I use the notebook to write absolutely everything I need to write down. And I write in it all messy—the messier the better: upside-down, sideways, in tiny script or big. I put everything in it: the name of a book you tell me about. A movie. The number of the plumber someone recommended. A monumental thought. A dream. Info about an appointment I'm making on the phone. A grocery list. To-do lists. A major brain dump. Anything and everything.

There is no order of importance to what I write in my notebook. My aim in a day is to write down everything I need to remember in my notebook. Everything!

So, part of the habit of using my notebook is to always be able to grab it—wherever I am.

Which is why I have extended my *desk notebook* technology (LOL) to include a second, tiny, satellite *desk notebook*. To be clear: I always have my main, medium-sized notebook nearby on my desk (or the couch or my bed) where I can grab it. But I have a second, lightweight, small *desk notebook* (mine is about 3-inch by 4.5-inch) in my pocketbook, backpack, or back pocket (if I'm out for a walk and inspiration, or anxiety, hits and I need to write something down).

Even if you use other tech for capturing info sometimes—having Siri take a note while you're driving, using your phone's camera to take a photo of something in a magazine, book, or online, etc., I think it's really important to gather all that information back into your main notebook at the end of the day.

Conversely, when I check in with my notebooks, I cross off things I don't need anymore, add something to an item I've already written, and transfer info to more permanent locations, like a paper or phone/computer contacts app, or calendar.

But even if you never transfer any information from your notebook to more long-lasting places, you'll always be able to go back to your notebooks and search around and find the name of that plumber somebody recommended.

I know a lot of people with ADHD can't keep track of a notebook, but I've learned to. I think this is a worthwhile hack to really try to master.

Notes App
(on Apple Devices)

I know I've just said (and have been saying for years) that I use my notebook for jotting down absolutely everything and that using one single notebook to gather all your information is essential for it to work.

But I have to admit that I've strayed: I don't want to admit it, but it's true and it's working for me.

So ... **in addition to using my *desk notebook*, I use the *Notes* app on my phone in the same way that I use my notebook.**

It's a super-simple app on both my iPhone and my MacBook, and they sync with each other.

So if I'm typing along on my laptop, and I think of something, I can click on the *Notes* app and write it down.

Later, when I'm on my phone, I can see what I've written in the Notes app on my computer. Or I can add another thing to the app from my phone and later, when I'm on my computer, it will be there.

And, if I'm driving, I can say, "Hey Siri, take a note," and the computer voice will say "What do you want it to say?" And I'll say, "Tell Marin about what Kevin said about Staci." And Siri will repeat the note and say the phone has added that note.

You can make a new note for anything you want, but I have only about 10 of them—movies and books, poems, work invoices, and others, but I don't like having too many different notes. (I don't like having too many of anything: I get overwhelmed.)

Instead, I have an Everything note that I put almost everything in.

It's funny that I don't mind the chaos of so many things written in the one note, but I don't.

Like my *desk notebook*, my *Everything* note is filled with everything and anything I want to, well, take note of: someone's address; ideas; grocery items to remember; doctor's appointments; a friend's birthday; chores; my dreams; a new goal; anything at all.

Later, I erase stuff, and move info to more permanent places, like my contacts or calendar apps or paper versions of same.

I don't know the Android operating system, but I'm sure it's just as good and has a version of the *Notes* app. And there's *Google Keep*, too, which I think is similar and can be used with any operating system. Actually, there are dozens of amazing notes apps out there, but this Mac app is amazingly simple, and I love that about it.

Go figure.

Brain Dump (Clearing Your Cache and Resetting Your Cookies)

When I'm feeling particularly overwhelmed or stressed, doing a "brain dump" helps.

It's easy. I take my notebook and write down "Brain Dump" and the date.

Then I write down every single thing I can think of that I want to do, I'm worried about, I'm bothered by, I'm afraid of, I'm stressing over, I'm ashamed of, I regret. Big and little. Real or imagined. Likely to happen or a fantasy.

Take your time and get it all out, all of it, whatever it is.

Don't worry about grammar, punctuation, or being neat.

Writing all these things out is like giving someone else a heavy object to hold for you.

When you think you're done, sit for another five minutes and rack your brain for more stuff.

I've had brain dumps that had more than 100 things on them. The following is a little brain dump I did the other day…

- Do laundry more regularly.
- Write a screenplay.
- Be early for work.
- Bring tuna fish to food bank.
- Get a big analog clock with hands.
- Stop interrupting.
- Scrub the grime in the tracks of the glass sliders going to the deck.
- Learn how to grow sprouts.
- Eat more vegetables.
- Meditate for 1 minute more often.
- Start weight training.
- Telephone more people.
- Clean your closet.
- Wash the floor.
- Start walking.
- Remove the lining in your bag.
- Hang your sweaters.

When you pin down all your swirling thoughts and nagging awarenesses, it relieves you of the need to keep remembering them. Once a thought is nailed down in black and white, it's much less likely to keep swirling in your mind.

I like looking over a brain dump later. I cross things out, move items around, sometimes use colors to highlight the most important things.

You can also rewrite the list, dividing its items into Today, Next week, or Someday.

You can use the *Brain Dump* to transfer items to your *to-do list*.

I always feel better when I get it all out of my head and onto paper.

Pros and Cons List

The good old pros and cons list is such a useful thing.

It's as simple as pie and about as solid a decision-making tool as pie is a solid dessert choice!

Say it's a decision whether to go to Los Angeles on vacation, or to New Orleans to see your mother. And man, you just cannot decide.

On a piece of paper, draw a line down the center vertically and one horizontally at the top of the page.

At the very top, write Trip Decision, and just under that, write pros on the left side of the vertical line, and cons on the right side.

Now, list all the pros of going to Los Angeles.

Then all the cons.

Do the same thing with New Orleans.

After you've really thought it through and written all the big and small pros and cons, you'll probably have a pretty good idea of which choice has the most pros.

You may think you know all these pros and cons, but often it isn't until you list them on paper that the weight of your pros and cons becomes clear.

Give it a try.

Your Own Digital Filing Cabinet

So, it's June 11, 2020, and we're 18 weeks or so into the virus, and it came out last week that people with Type A blood are likely to get much more seriously ill from Covid 19 than other blood types. (I believe this turned out to be untrue.)

And I think I have Type A blood, but I'm not sure, and I really want to know. **But where did I write down that information?**

I'm sure it's in one of my notebooks, but I have no idea what year I learned what my blood type was, and it would take hours to scour dozens of notebooks.

But guess what?

I opened the contacts app (the address book) on my phone and searched for "blood" like I would search for a person's name. And up came a contact named "Blood Type." And in the notes section at the bottom of its address card window, I had written A Positive.

Do you see what I do?

I store really important information in my address book just like it was a filing cabinet! Instead of putting in a person's name, I put in the bit of information I want to store.

I think it's the most fantastic idea, and I do it all the time!

Computer Bookmarks and Favorites Bars

I'm always trying to get my friends to "bookmark" the Internet pages on their web browsers they're interested in so they can go back to them with a single click.

And, I have to tell you, I can never talk anybody into doing it!

But I'm still going to tell you about them because I absolutely love using them. And maybe you will, too. They're such a useful way to organize information I want to remember or explore further.

If you're not familiar with bookmarking, it's choosing Internet pages to save as entries in a horizontal list called the Favorites or Bookmarks Bar, which runs along the top of your browser window on your computer.

You can bookmark anything—an article, a map, a store, someone's site—any page that you want to return to with a single click.

But *why I love bookmarking most*: You can also make a bookmark that's a *bookmark folder* that can store limitless bookmarks inside it. For instance, I have one that's labeled newspapers. And when I click on the newspapers bookmark folder, a dropdown menu has bookmarks to all the publications I normally read. This is hard to explain.

From a Mac Safari Internet search engine page, it's simple to make a bookmark or bookmark folder. All you have to do is:

- Click *Bookmarks* in the Safari menu that runs horizontally across the very top of your computer screen, to access its drop-down menu.
- Navigate to *Add Bookmark* or *Add Bookmark Folder* in the drop-down menu and click it.

You will then be prompted to choose where you want to save the new bookmark—either within an existing bookmark folder, or as an entry in the top-level list of *Favorites/Bookmarks*, and what to name it.

I give them short names, so I can fit lots of bookmarks along the top of my Safari window for easy access.

I make new bookmark folders a lot, and later if I don't want them, I just delete them.

For instance, I created a new bookmark folder in Safari a couple weeks ago and named it *garden*.

A few days later, when I was reading about how to grow Swiss chard, I bookmarked the page and saved it in the garden bookmark folder. Now the garden folder has about 15 saved pages—including ones on companion planting, using fencing, garden layout ideas, and lots more subjects.

Another example: When I go to a city, or on a trip, I make a folder for the trip or city. Then, as I research restaurants or anything interesting about the place, I bookmark those pages. Later, if I don't want the information anymore, I delete the folder.

All the search engines use bookmarking in both the Mac and Windows operating systems. The processes are a bit different, but it shouldn't be hard to learn how to use them.

Maybe you'll be the first person I've finally convinced to use them! (LOL).

Out of Sight, Out of Mind

Out of sight, out of mind works for me!

Sometimes I can't get started on something if the room, or my desk, is full of clutter. **Clutter is too much sensory input for me** because things snag my attention and make me want to do something about them. I do best in a simple space, free of miscellaneous stuff.

When my desk is a mess and I have to work, I sometimes take an empty crate and put everything in it, label it "desk junk Dec. 2020" and stash it out of sight. Having too much stuff around me attracts my attention and makes me anxious. And out of sight is largely out of mind with me, so it actually works.

The danger is never going back to retrieve it and having closets filled with boxes of clutter. But hopefully, you'll go back later and put things where they go. Or, if a year or so has passed and you haven't felt the need to go looking for something in the box, you could just throw it out.

It does sometimes hurt a little to give things away or throw them out, but mostly I love it because I feel so much better afterward!

Cleaning, Server-Style

Oh, I love cleaning (restaurant) server-style and letting myself fly from one thing to another!

If you've never worked as a server, you might not know what I'm talking about. Then again, if you have ADHD, you probably get the idea.

If you're a server and it's busy, you tear from one task to another ping-ponging among many tables, the kitchen, the bar, the bus station, the condiments station, the bread station… and back again!

You take an order, and on the way to post it to the kitchen, you pick up a dirty glass at another table, then swing two steps out of your way to grab bread for a third new table, head for the computer, put an order in, pick up another table's appetizers, deliver them, then drop the bread off at a table across the room. En route to get table four's entrees, you put in a drinks order at the bar, also filling a shot glass with several lemon wedges for a certain guest. And on and on it goes.

So, at home, it works similarly. Say I'm in the kitchen washing dishes when I remember that I need to fill a cosmetic-sized jar with coconut oil for use on my skin in the bathroom. I know I have just the right small glass jar and grab it from the cabinet, only to find that it has a bit of hardened honey stuck inside. So

I wash it and start to put it in the dish drain but see that the rack is filled with dry dishes, which I do not want to get wet by putting the now-clean, wet jar in on top of them (gawd!). So, I put the wet jar down on a kitchen cloth and start putting the dry dishes away and when I go to put some spoons in the drawer, I keep one instead, dry the jar, grab the coconut oil and head upstairs to the bathroom.

En route, I grab the bra—which I'd previously ripped off the minute I'd gotten home earlier in the day—and drop it off in my bureau. In the bathroom, I spoon out some coconut oil into the jar and put it away and see the nail clippers—so I clip my nails! Afterward, I drop the clippers off in the basket I keep nail polish stuff in, in the guest room closet, where I notice that the pillow cases are in a jumble, which I hate, so I take the pile out, and start folding.

And on and on it goes.

I wish I could remember the funny thing some woman posted on Instagram about her doing this kind of cleaning and somehow ending up naked in a football helmet and rubber boots with a spatula in her hand. (There's also another, old joke about a woman cleaning naked in a baseball hat, on a sweltering hot day, when the meter reader finds her in the basement and says "Jeeze, lady, I sure hope your team wins!")

Right?

Daily To-Do List (Staying Present to the Day's Needs)

"My parents didn't know about ADHD, but they intuitively understood me. And that's really what helped me to be as organized as I am—being able to stay on tasks—because they put certain things in place.

So, for example, keeping a calendar, right? My dad was really big on me having a planner—you know, putting things down—because he knew I forgot stuff. I forget everything, right? So for instance, this meeting here is in my planner. I also use Siri and set timers for appointments in my planner."

—Yakini, ADHDer, entrepreneur, and mother of two

A to-do list is an ongoing thing and part of what the old-school, paper planners (like Day Runners and Filofaxes) used to include.

I can't imagine staying remotely tethered to the planet if I didn't have the home plate of a to-do list to circle around.

If you're just beginning to use a to-do list, the most important thing is to keep the list in the same place all the time.

I put mine in my notebook because I always have it with me. I use fresh pages to copy it over each day. I cross stuff out and like allowing myself to make a big mess out of my pages.

It just makes sense to have a paper notebook and pen with you at all times, no matter how high-tech you are (and I actually am).

Scribbling on a page is still fast and easy.

I have my notebook in front of me for every phone call I make in case I want to write down something the other person says.

Either the night before, or in the morning of the day, I create my daily to-do list after looking through my notebook.

I just put about three to five items on my daily to-do list: And, if I haven't done the things from the day before, I move them onto to the new day's list.

Something like that.

A Way to Save Passwords

Okay: If you're an iPhone user, here's the easiest way to keep track of and protect your passwords.

Your iPhone comes with a *Notes* app. The app syncs with your computer, if you have a Mac.

You can create a new note for anything you want, and you can also lock notes.

So, I have one note that I keep locked. It can only be opened if I enter its password. And I created a weird password and memorized it. I put all my passwords in that one locked note.

Voila!

(**P.S. To do this, you absolutely have to remember the password to that one locked note.** Think hard, and maybe make it some short phrase or something funny…like RememberYourF*ckingPasswords, followed by three stars and your favorite color in lower case!

One Credit Card

Just use one credit card and one debit card.

Paying bills has always been a bitch for me. Even when I'm particularly flush: It's not even always about money worries: I just don't like anything about it and have a very hard time getting motivated. So who wants more credit card bills than they need? Forget about the 20 percent off you get to open a new credit card at a store, it's not worth it.

Just use one credit card—preferably one that gives you points—so you only have to pay one bill. Period.

Period.

Gift-Giving Hack

I have a hard time buying people presents. It's not that I'm mean, it's that I have a hard time thinking up what to buy them that's meaningful combined with a painful inability to decide among items. I'm guessing other unconscious (or undecided) things contribute to making it hard for me. Like how much money should I spend? And, not knowing if I have any wrapping paper, ribbon, and tape. Oh, and dreading having to write something monumental on the card so the person knows how much I love them.

Gift giving has always been a bit of a pressure situation for me.

But I'm happy to report that things are getting better in my gift giving department. Mostly, because I've finally begun to prepare for upcoming presenting times a little ahead of what has too often been a last-minute situation. Having the present wrapped and ready to go takes the stress out of the special day setting the stage for the possibility of joy. You're done! You can just suit up and show up because the gift part is DONE. You don't have to race out for wrapping paper, or worse, the gift itself.

So, what's helping me get started lately is to have created a little place where I keep the whole wrapping, carding, ribboning, things all together. Yes, Missy: I have a mini, portable wrapping station complete with pens, scissors, and tape!

(This sounds so tiny a thing to have to plan ahead but, hey: This is what it takes me to give a nice gift.)

Initially, I put all my gift-giving supplies in a box in a corner of a closet (with an old hardback book thrown in to keep the cards unwrinkled). But recently I bought a soft-sided, canvas, long, narrow, zippered case online. It was $20 and holds everything.

But the magic of the wrapping station only comes if you **always—and only—put your wrapping supplies in it.**

It makes giving presents much easier. It also promotes me giving tiny gifts for nothing—a jar of sea salt—more often, which is something I've always wanted to do.

So there!

F*ck it

> "My experience of life is too fun, varied, and interesting for me to care anymore about things looking a certain way. Post-it notes work the best this month? Who cares!
>
> It's not like my kitchen wall needs to look like an Instagram influencer's kitchen.
>
> The excitement I experience digging into a new passion interest is totally worth any perceived untidiness."
>
> —Gabi, (IG: @gabi_fisher)

A word here about a messy house.

While it's true that being organized makes doing lots of things easier, if you just can't do it sometimes, so what?!!

If the house is a mess, the house is a f*cking mess—it doesn't make you an axe murderer!

There's a point with all of our challenges where it's good to let go. Really. *If you can't, you can't. You're doing other things.*

I know a few women who are terribly disorganized and swing with it just the way it is. They don't apologize because their house is messy, or whatever, and they shouldn't.

Don't let the Marie Kondos of the world make it into a moral issue!

PART IV B

Time Management

Prepping Things

"Time has been something that I have struggled with: being on time for an event—time management in general.

At one point, I worked to identify why I was never on time and what I could do to correct it.

For instance, I noticed in the morning when leaving for work, **one thing that would constantly make me late was having to gather my lunch, bags, clothes, etc. Everything I needed for that day would be scattered all over the house which took a lot of time and even then** I'd usually wind up forgetting something on top of being late.

I now make sure everything is done the night before; I pack my lunch, put bags or whatever I need to bring and leave them by the door so they're ready to go in the morning.

Everything is about planning and preparation. If I had a doctor's appointment, in order to be on time, I would always make sure I allowed myself enough time for travel. However, I did not consider time for parking, walking/finding the office, traffic. So now I not only look up how long it will take to travel, but I also account for these other factors and try to allow myself extra time."

—Julie, physical therapist

Like Julie, I prep stuff in advance. Not only to avoid being late, but to avoid anxiety.

For instance, packing—for even just a weekend away.

I start getting ready a week or so ahead. It sounds geeky as heck, but it's the truth. If I don't do this, the prospect of having to do it hangs over me. And I hate that.

Typically, and it's funny, I start washing clothes even though I hate washing my clothes … bras, underpants, under tees, short sleeve tees, long sleeve tees—all the first layer stuff.

Then I get to washing the rest of my clothes and start thinking about what clothes and footwear I'm going to need or want to have to be good for the weather where I'm going and what I want to do when I'm there. **This isn't easy for me: I have to really think it through.**

I check my supplements and the meds I take, and make sure I have enough. I pack them in the containers I use for them, taking enough for the whole visit. I start packing my skin care and makeup bag a few days before leaving. I decide which suitcase(s) and get it/them out, maybe three days ahead.

You get the picture? You either really get the picture, or you can't believe how amazingly geeky I am. (And need to be.)

Other things I prep:

I have better days when I get dressed as soon as I get up. **Setting out my clothes the night before helps me put them on when I get out of bed.** (Doing this removes the whole layer of resistance I can have to getting dressed: *What am I going to wear?*)

Dinner (or **available food in the house**) when friends are coming over.

It totally helps me gather my thoughts and plan a meal by writing about it. I write with either a pen or a keyboard, either in my notebook or in my *Notes* app on my computer and iPhone.

I start with anything I'm thinking about the meal. **"Okay," I might write, "so they'll be six of us. Need a main course, two veggies, some light starch ... could use grapes or strawberries for dessert. Do I have to have appetizers? Ask Jane for ideas."**

If I can't think of what to make for a main course (even though I've made thousands of main courses in my life), I'll peruse my recipe bookmarks on my computer or my recipes folder on my computer.

What else? Can't remember!

Prioritizing What's Important

Too often, I spend time taking care of some BS task that urgently needs doing, right then, because I've blown off getting it done earlier.

It wasn't until I was diagnosed with ADHD that I understood that I'd never consciously established what I wanted most in life. I can thank my old therapist Jim for that awareness: It suddenly dawned on him, in one of our sessions, that I gave everything the same weight. "You can't tell the difference between what's really important to you, and what's not," he said.

From that point on, with his help, I learned to identify my priorities in life.

When you've identified your priorities, you have a throughline in your life that you can keep referring back to, to keep you on track.

I started with my lifetime priorities. What did I value and love most? On my death bed, what would I be proud and pleased to have done?

What's important to each of us is unique, but for me they're things that feed the soul: being a loving person; helping others; providing for your family; being a good parent, friend, relative;

strengthening your connection to something greater than yourself: developing faith in the good; nurturing your inner child; healing family of origin wounds.

From there, I learned to extrapolate daily priorities: Things I could work on in my daily life that were in sync with my lifetime priorities. Actions that I could take that would build up over a lifetime.

When I haven't established my priorities, I end up spending my days racing after something new or urgently catching up with tasks I've neglected.

The high energy of doing things urgently makes it feel like I'm accomplishing big things, but so often urgent things aren't important!

The late, great time management guru, Stephen Covey, was known for suggesting that people identify the difference between things in their lives that are important and things that are merely urgent—but not important.

I included the following story in my first book, and I'm going to include it here because it's so helpful in understanding what I'm trying to say:

No one seems to know where the story originated. I've read it in several places, including Covey's book, *First Things First*. In any case, it graphically illustrates how important priorities are and how daily priorities depend on having identified your big, lifetime priorities: those values, goals, and things that are most important to you.

So, the story goes that a teacher stands in front of his students with a big gallon-sized glass jar into which he places several large rocks until the jar can't take anymore. At that point, he asks the class if the jar is full.

"Yes, yes, of course," answer the students, at which point the smiling teacher pours in a few cups of smaller rocks, jiggling the jar until they have filled in the spaces around the large rocks. At that point, he again asks the class if the jar is full.

Suddenly hip to the teacher, they all say no. At which point, he pours some sand into the jar, which filters down and fills in the empty spaces among the big and small rocks. At that point he, again, asks the class if the jar is full. Knowing what they will answer, he begins filling the jar with water and asks again, if the jar is full. To which everybody yells, "Yes, it's full now!"

The moral: You've got to get your big rocks (most important things) in place first or you won't be able to fit them into your life.

Chunking

Say, you have to write a resume for yourself and you keep putting it off, but you really need one to get a job.

One of the big reasons why you're procrastinating is likely because you don't know where to start. But if you break the project down into several separate tasks, it will make it much, much easier.

This is called chunking. And it's especially helpful for ADHDers.

With the example of a resume, you might break the project down into the following chunks, or steps, which you can do one at a time:

- Research formats for resumes.

- There are lots of examples online of different ways you can organize and present information about yourself in a resume. Search the Internet for sites on "how to write a resume." If you have experience in a couple different fields of work, write a resume for each field, so you can emphasize the pertinent parts of your experience in that field and leave out other stuff.

- Spend some time reading sample resumes. Reading sample resumes is likely to spark your interest and give you some ideas about how you want to structure yours. Take notes about what you like.

- Decide which style you're going to emulate for your resume. You may even mix and match parts of different resume styles to suit your particular assets. Take a piece of paper and sketch out a mock resume in the style you're going to follow.

- Gather all the facts you can about your previous jobs so you have the dates (approximate dates are fine) and proper names all spelled correctly. Gather your educational info. If you didn't finish a degree, you should still list "UCLA 1992-4." Also include any special training you've had, like Course work, Harvard University, Technical Editing.

- Gather info on any special skills you may have, like the software programs you're fluent in, languages you speak, that you're a people-person who excels at interpersonal relationships. Go review the websites on resumes again and see how others have done this. Copy their style (never their exact words).

- If you're stuck on any part of the resume writing, get some help. Talking with a friend about it might help you get a clearer idea about what you know but can't access alone.

Having completed these different chunks, put the whole thing together on your computer. If you can't format it well, hire a freelancer on Upwork.com or another freelance job site to type it properly for you.

Finally, go over every single letter and word and space in the final document, looking for typos and correct them.

Then do that again.

There's always another typo! Keep looking!

Transitioning

Transitioning from one task to another is hard for a lot of people with ADHD.

You know how it is: **Sometimes you just can't get motivated to do something you're not interested in and other times you're so deeply interested in something that you just don't want to stop.**

As we've said before, **the name Attention Deficit Hyperactivity Disorder is misleading because it's not that we lack attention, it's that we can't always deploy our attention *on demand*.** Our attention is intense—it gets so deeply engaged, when it's engaged, that it's very difficult to withdraw.

But life often demands a more fluid type of attention that can be switched off and on more easily.

Acknowledging what's required when transitioning from one task to the next will help you become better at doing this.

Transitioning requires at least two major mental muscles (they're actually considered executive functions).

The first is the ability to inhibit ourselves by withdrawing our interest in something mid-stream (your boss walks in with a last-minute rush job).

The second is shifting our interest to a new task.

Both withdrawing interest and deploying it to something new are characteristically challenging efforts for ADHDers, so we need strategies to accomplish both of them.

Stopping abruptly and jumping into some physical activity right away often works for me as a first step to withdrawing attention.

Depending on the situation, you can **create a habitual physical movement to give yourself time to adjust from one focus to another**: If you're **at work**, you might **go to the bathroom**, to the **coffee station**, or the **water cooler**. If you're **at home**, you can do any number of things like **jumping on an exercise machine for a minute**, just **jumping in place**, **going outside**, or some other action.

Once you've detached from what you'd been focused on, you're going to need to bend your focus to the new thing with which you need to engage.

You can do this with the help of any number of strategies you're already using:

- **Set a timer** for eight minutes and tell yourself you only have to engage for eight minutes (usually, by the time the timer goes off, you've started and become engaged).
- **Blast a piece of music** that puts you in the zone and ride that stimulation into the first few minutes of the new task.
- **Glance at your notebook**, Post-its, or whiteboard where you can read your goals again and reacquaint yourself with them.
- You can **text your coach or ADHD friend** that you're doing it—you're transitioning!

If you can foresee the different tasks, you'll be required to do in a given time period, **it will help you get started if you've set out some of the tools you're going to need for the new task ahead of time.**

Like, if it's an email that has to be returned, forward the email to yourself so it's at the top of your email list. If it's vacuuming, set out the vacuum cleaner. If it's going to a work meeting, set out your notebook, pens, and whatever else you'll need in the meeting. If it's paying bills, go touch the pile of papers: Just touch it.

All of these things help me transition from one intense activity to the next.

Analog Clocks

There is such time blindness in some women with ADHD that experts liken it to a nearsighted person's poor vision. Many of us can't judge time well and the only time that is really vivid to us is NOW.

One of the many strategies for becoming more aware of time is to use analog clocks and watches. The hour, minute, and second hands help us visualize time passing better than looking at a digital readout, which just displays 11:11 a.m., for instance.

That's it: Get an analog clock with regular old-school hands.

You can never have too many wall clocks, either (try the Dollar Store).

Big Whiteboard

Plenty of ADHDers, no matter how smart they are, can't consistently use a notebook, datebook, calendar, or computer app for keeping themselves on task.

We'll start to use one and maybe keep up with it for a period of time, then stop.

Sometimes we stop because we simply change our minds and don't think it's a good idea anymore. **Sometimes** it's because we feel a tremendous resistance to going back to that same boring method. **Sometimes** it's because we think a new app or notebook or organizing system will be better and we go after that. And yet other times, it's because we lose track of where a notebook is, or which app it was we were using, and it all becomes a blur.

But a big whiteboard that's right there in front of you is much harder to ignore or forget.

If you have room for one, I highly recommend it.

Use it any which way you can and **make it your own.**

Glue a couple colored pens to some string and somehow attach them to the board, so you can easily grab one and jot down whatever you want.

Erase items and **rewrite them** in another part of the board.

Move info from the board to another more secure location.

Consult what's written there when you're making a daily to-do list.

Draw a picture of a big smiling face on the board, or a tape up a picture of yourself, or someone you love or admire.

Try to love the big whiteboard by continuing to go back to it, refresh it, decorate it, use different pens, surround it with icons or mementos you love. Give it your own special ZHUZH!

Jot Everything Down

If you're doing something and then, out of nowhere, suddenly feel like you absolutely have to know how to dye your leather bag blue or what time of the year to plant roses, writing those things down can help you avoid getting distracted and going after them.

Jotting things down can assuage the impulse to go after a passing attraction right that minute.

Jotting something down, where you know you'll be able to find it later, can relieve that strong desire to go after it now.

Jotting it down is like giving it to a friend to hold: You know it's safe and that you can get to it later.

It works for me quite a bit of the time.

Scheduling

I've always been very resistant to committing to a weekly event: a class, a date, a party, *anything*. I so hate to commit! And often when I do, I dread having to do the thing all week long. Luckily, when I finally go to the event—whatever it is—I generally have a good time. But what a pain in the ass!

Meanwhile, for the past 18 months, I've been going to the same five Zoom group meetings every single week.

And I can't tell you how helpful this has been for me! For some reason, a few months after those five time slots were set in stone, it became easier to schedule other tasks around them.

Now, I have several other things I do at the same time each week. After one of my two classes, I grocery shop because the class is near Trader Joe's. After the other class, I hit Whole Foods.

These repeating commitments help ground me. They're like tethers that anchor me as time flies by.

Routine, it turns out, is reassuring. And it makes it so, so much easier to get things done than having to go through the whole rigamarole of finding a good time to do this, that, or the other thing.

Routine events become habitual and once a habit is established, whatever it is, things become easier to do.

Not only does scheduling routine events help me get things done, but the leftover chunks of time have made it easier for me to see when I can slot in other activities.

Obviously, I'm not reinventing the wheel here. Doing things at the same time every week is how much of society operates, you know: 9-5 and all that. But for me, it's new and revelatory!

My Beloved Timer Tool

I have a lot of trouble starting things I don't want to do.

(The dishes come to mind. They are f*cking constant. Every single day even if I hardly cook—if I just make sandwiches or eat leftovers or make a small salad—dishes, dishes, dishes!)

Because getting started is one of the most painful parts of my ADHD, I have to use a lot of strategies to get going.

One of my favorites is to use a timer. Maybe you know about it, but I'll tell you anyway.

If I'm in the kitchen and it's a mess, and I really do not want to dive in there but I know (from experience) how good it'll feel to have a clean sink in the morning, I set the oven timer to eight minutes.

Of course, you can use any smallish number of minutes you want, but I seem to have become attached to the number eight.

And I start cleaning.

If there are any dishes in the drain rack, I put them away first so I will have somewhere to put the newly washed dishes. Then I start washing them.

Once I get going, I usually get into it.

I know I only have to do it for eight minutes.

Turns out you can get a lot of dishes done in eight minutes, and I often finish. But if I don't, I stop washing because I know I promised myself I only had to do it for eight minutes.

If I'm not finished, but I want to finish, I set the alarm again, maybe for only three minutes. Or another eight if there's a lot to do, and I feel like I don't mind doing it. And then I finish.

If, however, I'm not finished when the timer goes off and I don't feel like continuing, I stop. And things won't be all neat and clean, but they'll be closer to getting there. And I will have accomplished something!

I can't recommend the timer method enough. If you get into it, you might want a good timer that's easy to use. A lot of people use their phones. But you might want to have a watch timer so it's always right there *on you*. I ended up getting an Apple Watch, because it's easy to use the timer. (I got an older used model on Craigslist. All I really wanted was the timer.)

PART IV C
Self-Knowledge

Self-Inventory

"Working with my ADHD has been a part of my life for a long time. I was able to manage it initially without medication, then with medication, then with medication and school accommodations, then finally I discontinued medication altogether.

I think today, the one thing that helps me manage the most is self-reflection and really identifying specifically how ADHD affects my life *and then consciously modifying my behavior in order to maintain some control over how I live my life."*

—Julie, physical therapist

You know that frustrating state you can find yourself in when you know you should be able to do a thing, you promised yourself you would, you were so excited about doing it the other evening, but right now when it needs doing—**you just can't lift a f*cking finger?**

Not being able to get motivated to start something is tough stuff.

Understanding some of the science behind our difficulties getting motivated is reassuring, but we're still left with the job of having to find **how to break through and get started.**

Self examination, like Julie said above, is one of the most useful ways.

ADHD expert William Dodson, M.D., thinks **the most powerful thing you can do when you have ADHD is to figure out** *precisely what situations and environments turn you on,* which is why he recommends that people with ADHD compile a written self-inventory.

Once you become aware of the different activities and environments that stimulate you, you can use one of them to jump-start your engine, so to speak, *and then use that energy to coast into the designated task.*

To find out what triggers you into a stimulated state, Dodson has people keep a notebook for a month and write down every situation in which they're thriving and succeeding in their real lives.

Do you feel up and motivated after being with a close friend? Do you feel energized after finishing work? After a walk? A yoga class? How about after learning something entirely new on the Web? Are you motivated in group situations, like working with a partner? When you're competing with others? In a leadership position? Do you only do your very best on a deadline? In a totally quiet room? Or with music you love blaring?

In a July 2021 article in ADDitude Magazine, William Dodson talks about ADHDers' success using this self-inventory:

"At the end of the month, most people have compiled 50 or 60 different techniques that they know work for them. When called on to perform and become engaged, they now understand how their nervous system works and which techniques are helpful.

"I have seen these strategies work for many individuals with ADHD, because they stepped back and figured out the triggers they need to pull. This approach does not try to change people with an ADHD nervous system into neurotypical people (as if that were possible) but gives lifelong help because it builds on their strengths."

Talking Nice About All Our Brains

Just like some of us are great at drawing and lousy at organizing, or good at imitating accents but poor at decision making, each of our brains is good at some things and has trouble with others.

Talking about what our brains have trouble with and what they're good at is a terrific, much-needed way to destigmatize ADHD. It's also a great way to begin to see and capitalize on the assets that are as much a part of ADHD as its well-known (half-understood) challenges!

The wonderful writer Sarah Wheeler wrote a piece on her Momspreading blog about how she talks to kids—her own and others in her practice as a child psychologist—about all our different brains. It seems so obvious a thing to do and yet I don't think it's entered the popular culture yet.

"Hey, buddy," she might say to a kid, "my brain loves looking for lost Lego pieces, but has a hard time building them, what about your brain? Do you like looking for them or building them more?"

Using yourself as an example and sharing what your brain is good at and what it struggles with is the perfect missing link in the neurodiversity movement! **Let's get these conversations started!**

Excavate Your Authentic Self, Part 1: How We May Have Lost Ourselves

I recently saw an old video of a friend's wedding reception. One short segment was of me talking with some people. Watching it reminded me vividly of what I was doing and feeling in that moment so many years ago. I wasn't just there, being myself, enjoying the present moment: No, I was occupied feeling several other people's discomfort and busy saying things to draw them into conversation, make them feel welcome, and, to be painfully honest, communicate to them that I was a nice person.

This is an example of a caretaking behavior stemming from the mistaken notion that I should be what other people want me to be. If you dig deeply into this behavior, you'll find **people-pleasing** woven into the mix.

For me, it evolved in childhood—living with a verbally abusive father. To try to stop him from exploding, I said things to appease him.

And in order to know what to say to derail him from blowing up, I had to be riveted to his moods. And to be riveted to another person's moods, you have to shut down your own emotional needs. I didn't know this at the time, but I've since learned a lot about it.

When growing up, **many women with ADHD enact a very similar abandoning of themselves in order to fit into a culture that doesn't accommodate their differences.**

Surrounded by a society—adults, parents, teachers—who are ignorant about the ADHD brain and blind to its needs and assets, many of us grow up being criticized.

And, **to avoid attracting this painful criticism, we learned to try to appear "normal." And to learn how to do that, we studied other women so we could emulate their behavior.**

Spending your awareness studying neurotypical people so you can act like them and fit in requires that you abandon your connection to your own feelings and needs.

All of which amounts to losing a lot of yourself: If you're constantly tuned into other people's feelings, how can you possibly tune into your own? You can't, because emotionally and cognitively you're otherwise occupied.

This constant vigilance puts you in an energetic place where you aren't present within yourself—feeling your own feelings.

No: You're tuned into others, to make sure you can respond to them appropriately so they will think you're okay.

Years of emotionally abandoning yourself like this leaves a lot of women with ADHD not knowing what they feel; what they like; what they do not, in fact, like; and where they stand on different issues!

See the next entry for some ways to reconnect to your head and heart and begin to reclaim your authentic self.

Excavate Your Authentic Self, Part 2: What You Like, What You Don't Like, and More

What if who I am today is exactly who I'm supposed to be?

I've given up on personal development—as an ADHDer, it always seemed to end up as a pursuit to turn myself into a neurotypical person.

So these days, I assume I'm working on the "right" things, that I'm already who I'm supposed to be, and maybe all of that is exactly what the world needs.

—Gabi (IG: @gabi_fisher)

In the previous entry, I shared what happens to many women with ADHD that causes us to be out of touch with our authentic selves: with what we like, don't like, feel, don't feel, want, don't want.

I feel like I was drop-kicked out of the womb into life and raced ahead blindly in a purely reactive mode—rejecting or complying—with the adult influences around me. Looking back, I don't think I really knew what I genuinely felt or liked until I was in my 30s.

This happens to a lot of people and is likely even more prevalent in women with ADHD.

Below are some of the ways you can begin to reclaim your authenticity and discover where you stand, what your dreams are, what you like, what you want, and what you feel.

Excavating your authentic self can't be done in a day, but you can start on it in a day. And, since you're reading this, I suspect that you're already on the road.

I know I'm word-oriented, so I do this kind of exploring on paper, in my notebook or journal, so I can look back at it. But you could do it into the recorder on your phone or by drawing pictures as you ponder some of the following questions:

What am I good at?

What would I say if someone asked me, "What's the truth about you?"

If I weren't afraid, I would (fill in the blank).

Who do I really admire? Why?

What do I believe is my most beautiful quality?

If money weren't an issue, I would (fill in the blank).

If I could receive assistance from a Higher Power (God, the Universe, Spirit, friends, helpers), what would I ask for?

As you go through this exploration, you might notice negative thoughts flying through your head. They're just stuff our minds have picked up and *they can't be trusted*. They're a shitty part of the human condition (in my opinion), and comprise what the therapist and mindfulness meditation teacher Tara Brach calls our "trances of unworthiness."

I believe that the only thing these critical thoughts are good for is tipping you off to where you need to do some work. In other words, if a thought comes that says "I'm not good at anything," you can start turning that around by using an affirmation like, "I'm good at many things," or "I'm a warm, loving person," or "I love that I think deeply about life," or "I am honest with myself" or "It's safe to see all the good in me."

Helping comfort and **dismantle the critical inner self** that all people have is key to excavating our authentic selves.

As a woman with ADHD, I'm guessing you're very compassionate. Try applying that same compassion you have for others to yourself.

I love eccentric, different people. There's pretty much nothing I love more than women who show who they are to the world: authentic women who feel free to dance to their own unique drummers!

Dwell on the Good

According to psychologist Rick Hanson, author of the New York Times bestseller *Hardwiring Happiness: The New Brain Science of Contentment, Calm, and Confidence*, our brains lay down neural patterns rapidly when negative events happen.

To be clear: When something bad happens to us, our brains (somehow) physically embed thoughts of the event in neural pathways in our gray matter. **Negative events make a big impression on us so we can recognize the same danger very quickly the next time** we see it.

Our ancestors' brains evolved this way to survive: If dangers didn't make a big impression on them, they could perish (because they might not recognize particular dangers fast enough the next time).

And our brains still behave this way.

On the other hand, good things happen all the time—from the merely pleasant to the powerfully good—**but they don't make as big an impression on our brains.** Something great happens, but unless it's on the scale of a massive lottery win or relief after a cancer scare, the good thing doesn't stay with us long. We're happy about it, but we quickly move on.

To counter this, and lay down positive neural pathways that will help us experience positive emotions more quickly in the future, **Hanson recommends savoring the positive.**

When something good happens, says Hanson, don't just let it pass. **Dwell on the positive experience, for 30 seconds at least, focusing on how nice it feels: how happy you are that it happened.**

Hardwiring happiness like this will cue your brain to lay down neural pathways of positive feelings and ultimately help you feel good more of the time.

Let Go of Perfection

Lately—it's five weeks into our quarantine—I'm having a hard time making myself exercise.

And, for once, I'm not crucifying myself for feeling lazy. This pandemic is a trauma for all of us, and I think it's totally okay if I feel like I can't do much some days. This massive world change is a lot for the human psyche to integrate.

Still, a thought just drifted through my head saying, "wouldn't it be nice to come out of this quarantine stronger than I went in?"

So … even though there's no way I have the motivation to walk five miles a day like my sister, I can still do *something*, right?

So I went for **a short walk** today in the sunshine. And just now I did **five minutes of yoga.** And that was a nice effort for me under the circumstances. Dropping my desire to do an hour workout allowed me to start exercising, rather than stay stuck on the couch.

Perfection doesn't exist, yet the ADHD mind can get so hyperfocused on an effort that it keeps digging to find the absolutely best way to approach this, that, or the other thing.

Relentlessly digging for the perfect thing will eventually tire you out and from there you'll probably just abandon the whole effort.

The key to taking action is to decide on something that's good enough: something within your grasp and available, possible, affordable, or understandable.

Digging for the perfect thing—employment, a recipe, jacket, or therapist—**keeps you stuck,** not moving forward with what it is you want to do.

Once you let the good be good enough, you'll be able to move forward and actually do whatever it is you've been trying to do.

Allow Grace

Say you're stopped at a light or street corner, and an idea about how you can change your employment in a way that will really make things much better just suddenly pops into your head.

You've wanted to quit cigarettes for ages, and one day you just don't want to smoke anymore.

You're lonely and someone you come to love moves in a couple doors down.

You wish so much that you were part of a women's group of some sort, and a woman at your local cafe mentions that she goes to one. You've had neck pain for six months, and you suddenly realize it's gone.

This is Grace. The freely-given, creative unfolding of life in a positive direction *that just comes*. It's endless, really, if you want to trip out on the concept. Think of the sun. The air. The encounter with someone who mentions a remedy you've never heard of for an issue you have.

Good things proceed from the invisible realm all the time, but we sometimes push so hard we don't have room *to allow good to come in*.

Our culture definitely values the idea of trying really hard. And it's good to try hard. But sometimes you can try too hard. You push and push and push for something you have in mind, but it isn't working.

In cases like this, why not fall back and practice allowing whatever it is to just be?

Develop Your Observer

Instead of believing every critical thought your mind throws at you—about how deficient you are—maybe consider the idea that these critical thoughts are not true.

Researchers estimate that nearly 6,000 thoughts fly through the average mind each day.

Many of these thoughts are self-critical or otherwise negative, and they whack away at us, zapping our vital energy, depressing us, and twisting us into people who think we're not good enough.

This seems to be a massive human problem. I know it is for me.

Lots of good teachings are based on the idea that many of our thoughts are not to be trusted.

Self-help speaker and writer Byron Katie's therapeutic work is based on the idea that we aren't our thoughts. Working with individuals, she takes that basic premise and begins questioning people's negative beliefs about themselves.

Even if you don't get into Katie's work, **you can start to get some separation from your self-debasing thoughts just by becoming aware of them.**

Using part of your mind as a non-judgmental Observer of your thoughts is one way to go deeper here. It's a *meta-awareness—awareness of your awareness!*

After having decided that you're going to try to catch negative thoughts as they occur, you watch for them. And when you catch one ("I'm a really lousy neighbor. I never ask them over and they know it"), you take a minute to observe the thought occurring.

You can use this meta-awareness, aka non-judgmental observer, in so many sticky situations.

In the above case, I would pause, withdraw into my Observer, and acknowledge what was happening: "My mind is entertaining BS thoughts full of old tapes that might have protected me from something once, but I don't need anymore," I might say to myself.

And that moment of observing the thoughts in my mind can create a little space between me and my thoughts. And from the respite of that little space, I may be able to leave the thoughts behind and move on.

The concept of the non-judgmental Observer comes from various self-realization practices.

The non-judgmental Observer doesn't judge anything as good or bad, its job is just to observe what's happening.

I've heard it said that people in India train elephants to stop thrashing their trunks around by giving them a stick to hold.

Using a moment of your Observer acts to calm the racing mind like the stick calms the thrashing elephant.

After doing this for a while, your Observer will pop into your head more readily as you go through your day.

Tiny Gratitude List

Just think of three things you appreciate about the day you just had. (It's May 29, 2020, and the virus is still going strong.)

Focusing on what you appreciate is transformative and can actually draw more things to you that you appreciate.

How?

Like attracts like. (Birds of a feather flock together!)

So, just three things.

I'll go here:

That I learned how to make chicken wire "covers" for my garden to protect the plants from rabbits and deer.

That I took a walk.

That I have a roof over my head and the freedom (money) to buy food and my other needs.

Use a Journal

It's so hard to track specific troublesome aspects of ADHD because it comprises so many parts, the mind is infinitely complex, life is a mystery, and each of us is unique!

Because of all this, a big difficulty a lot of women with ADHD have is a general sense of confusion and overwhelm: **Should I do *this*? Should I do *that*? Oh, shit, I *have* to do this! Oh shit, I have to do *that*, and *that*, and *that*, and *THAT*!**

Writing in a journal helps us recognize what's on our minds and relieves anxiety by identifying issues, in concrete terms, and sets them apart from everything else. Writing something down sets it in stone and puts a spotlight on it.

Whether it's something that's happened or that I'm thinking about, worried about, happy about, or confused by, **writing about it relieves me of having to keep that particular thing in mind.**

It's also freeing to let your journal be messy—both in penmanship and the sense your sentences make. (Absolutely forget grammar!) Let yourself fly around, commenting any way you want about things that happened or that you've been thinking, doing, experiencing, whatever. **Here's the start of what I wrote the other day:**

"I sent Ande a long email about how Edith's doing. It felt good. I've loved the sun today. Took myself to the café at 4 just to see some people and have a coffee as a special treat because I felt a little lonely. That perked me up just enough to call Jane (look into cheaper Duette type window shades.) Connecting with Jane lifted my spirits, although I notice that sometimes on the phone with people I feel anxious when there's a pause ... you know, like a silence for a few seconds. That's nuts, isn't it? WTF? My sister Toni and I are a riot when we talk on the phone: Not only are there never any silences, but we go so far as to talk over each other, sometimes both talking full sentences at the same time with neither one of us backing down! I know it's not great but I love that we allow ourselves to do this! We hang up really abruptly, too. All it takes is one of us to say "gotta go"—even in the middle of something—and the other instantaneously says "bye" and hangs up."

There's a great writing teacher, Natalie Goldberg, who recommends that you start journaling by designating how many minutes you're going to write or how many pages you're going to fill.

After that, you put the pen to the paper, and *you never stop moving it until you're done.* Doing this makes you keep writing, sometimes goofy stuff ("I don't know what to say here ... I'm moving the pen"), but often something deep and important comes out. She's wonderfully inspirational about the value of journaling and has lots of exercises and prompts in her book, *Writing Down the Bones.* (I'm guessing Julia Cameron's "morning pages," in her book The Artist's Way, evolved from Goldberg's work.)

Anyway, my point is that on days that I've written in my journal, I feel way better. I feel less burdened and less overwhelmed. Sometimes, later in the day after having written, I feel like I do after having gone to (talking) therapy. In a good way: I feel somehow caught up, emotionally. It's a grounded feeling.

Consider a Digital Journal (If You Change Your Mind About a Paper One)

As I said in the last entry, I find it seriously therapeutic to have **a place to write whatever I want, to myself, in the total privacy of my own head.**

It's simple: *You just write anything that's on your mind—**from the most intense, life-altering stuff to the most meaningless fluff.** In a private place for your consumption only.*

Meanwhile, though, for quite a few years, I haven't liked writing long-hand anymore! I have tried, unsuccessfully, to talk myself into consistently using my current paper journal but I just haven't wanted to. I really prefer typing. I type fast, which is kind of fun in and of itself. (I don't have to look if I don't want to.)

So during this last bunch of years when I've been writing less frequently in my paper journal, I've also been typing journal pages in MS Word on my computer. But these pages are pretty unorganized and their state of dispersal, all over my hard drive, makes me anxious.

Because of this, for a while I was stuck between longhand journaling in a paper journal and typing journal entries in Word documents.

Until I finally got unstuck and admitted that I wasn't going to have a beautiful paper diary anymore and that I should embrace using a computer diary, and I have!

I've ended up with *Day One*, and I like it. It's super simple, secure, and it syncs between my computer and my phone so I can write in it either on my laptop or on my cell. I also really like that it has the date on each new entry, the location, and the weather.

An added bonus is that when using it on your phone you can hit the microphone and dictate instead of using your thumbs.

What if you wrote a few sentences a day, every day?

Best Environments for You

Soon after the virus hit, in March 2020, **I got an email from a woman** who wrote to say she'd liked my first book. It felt great to connect with her, and we wrote back and forth a couple times. She is a psychologist and included a link to a great blog post she'd just written.

Her post was about how **she'd always thought that being an extrovert was better than being an introvert.**

Then she suddenly realized that in a quarantine situation, it was better to be introverted.

And from that experience, she understood **how very supportive the right environment is for a particular individual's nature.**

I have a friend who always sits in the front row to help her pay attention.

I can't write with music on in the background, but my niece, Ally, does better work with something audible blaring.

Some people hate living on a noisy street, and some love the feeling of connection that the noise of a lively neighborhood gives them.

Do you like your toys/tools all around you when you work, or prefer a perfectly clear desktop?

Do you learn best by listening, or reading?

What time of day is your most energetic? What time the calmest?

Keep a list of this simple inventory of the environments that help you get motivated and hang the paper up where you can see it.

PART IV D
Self Care

Not So Hard! (What Stress is and Does to Us)

I don't know if I wrote about this in my first book, but I'll never forget it, so I'm going to mention it again here.

I was at my friend's house talking. We'd just had some lunch and she was wiping down her kitchen counter. And suddenly, I realized how hard she was scrubbing: She was pressing the sponge into the countertop with much more force than she needed to get the job done. And I got hysterical laughing because I saw so clearly how so many of us do so much with more stress and strain than we need to.

I catch myself throughout the day doing the simplest things hard: I mean hard as in *expending way more anxiety and energy than is needed to do the task*. When I catch myself, I have to make a big effort to slow down, calm down, take a few deep breaths, and try to come into the present moment.

Doing everything hard stems from a general anxiety I have that's often fueled by a crushing awareness that I have so many other things to do and want to do—and feeling that everything can only be done right away. It's a grinding pressure I feel because I sense that now is the only time there is. It's that ADHD internal race-car brain that just wants to go, go, go.

Not only does this state of mind hurt my mind-body, but it prevents me from being in the present! *I'm washing dishes: Water—this magical life-giving substance—is flowing from a faucet. This is now. There's nowhere else to go: I'm here. Calm down. Breathe.*

And what it all amounts to is stress: It's low-level stress, but it's chronic stress, nonetheless. And although we toss around the word stress as though it were nothing much, **stress is, in fact, an actual physiological state in the body that is corrosive and debilitating.**

The stress response, aka fight or flight, evolved when humans needed extra energy to take care of life-threatening situations. This ancient coding floods the body with adrenaline and cortisol and other stress compounds and hormones that give us momentary boosts of energy so we can do super-human things.

When we're stressed, our hearts immediately begin to beat faster, our blood pressure rises, stored blood sugar and fat are released, and dozens of stress hormones and substances flood the body. These and other changes give our brains more oxygen and our muscles more strength so our senses sharpen and our bodies become more powerful.

Meanwhile, though, to create all this instant energy means the body withdraws energy from all the regular, ongoing, routine, maintenance functions we continuously undertake to keep us alive and healthy: **We stop repairing cells, eliminating waste, managing body heat, digesting food, patrolling for foreign invaders (what our immune system does), and much, much more.**

All of which is to say that chronic stress depletes our bodies and minds in untold ways and leads to a range of very real illnesses.

The fight-or-flight response is still ready, today, to kick in to help us in disasters or dangerous situations, which is great.

But the problem is that all too often our bodies and minds leap into terror or anxiety over things that are not critical to our survival. Consequently, most of us spend much more time in a stressed state than we have to. I know I do!

My hope is that knowing that stress is an actual (slow) killer will not only heighten our awareness of it but also motivate us to seek out ways to calm ourselves down as often as we can.

One Push Up

I had a hilarious dream last night (July 2021). It was that I was with a woman who lived in a glass house. Even the ceiling was glass. And—because in real life I live in a house with a lot of (usually dirty) windows—I asked her how she could possibly keep all her windows clean.

"We do two a day," she said!

I try to do things this way: a little bit at a time, relaxed and confident in the truth that each little bit adds up.

I love the story of this guy Stephen Guise, who wrote the book *Smaller Habits, Bigger Results*. It's about how he finally, after years of being unable to stick with any workout routine became a worker-outer! How? **He set the goal for himself of doing ONE PUSH-UP A DAY.**

He'd spent 10 years wanting and failing to motivate himself to get in shape. None of the regular strategies worked for him. And one day, so frustrated by his inability to do his 30-minute workout, he asked himself what the opposite of a strenuous 30-minute workout was? And he came up with the idea of doing one single push-up.

So he started doing one push-up a day. That was his only goal: a goal that required so little willpower that he figured he could stick with it. And he did.

I love this and think it's profound. **Doing your one little thing, day after day, generates a tiny bit of power (fulfillment/reward/happy brain chemicals), which is enough to fuel you to do it again!**

I know you're thinking: Right. One f*cking push-up? One lousy push-up won't get me anywhere. It'll take too long to amount to anything. I want the whole thing now!

But what Guise found was that once he was down there, doing his one push-up, he felt like doing another.

As they say, there is more than one way to skin a cat!

Can you choose one mini-habit to commit to doing every day?

Here are some ideas:

- Driving to the gym, walking inside, touching a treadmill, and going home.
- Putting your pajamas away in the same place every morning.
- Making your bed when you get up.
- Writing down one thing you're grateful for in the same small gratitude notebook you keep in the same place, every night.
- Doing one push-up, downward dog, plank, or other single exercise you know is good for you.

Forest Bathing

I like this newish idea out there even though it's kind of a trendy, commercialized take on the most natural thing. Have you heard of it? Forest bathing.

From what I'm reading, **it started in Japan where the government has preserved dozens of forests throughout the country so people can go to them and walk, sit around in and yes, bathe, in a natural, not man-made environment.**

Numerous studies have shown the health benefits of just being outside—the greener, the better. **Going outdoors reduces a range of stress markers which, in turn, enhances our ability to regulate ourselves.**

I don't have to read these studies to know how good it is for me to be outside, I can feel it. Especially in the winter here in the Northeast. Any amount of time outside is restorative in the most real way.

And I don't take my f*cking phone. (We're getting hammered by our (fabulous) phones, IMO. I am anyway.)

Clearly, human beings are part of nature and connecting with it resets us in a healthy way.

Just 20 minutes outside can calm us down, fortifying our exhausted executive functions by resting and resetting our brains.

Which doesn't mean that only two minutes outside doesn't help us. It does. **Any amount of time spent outdoors helps reset us to our factory settings.**

Parks, cemeteries, oceans, lakes, streams and rivers, patches of undeveloped land ... no matter where you are, I hope you start to go outside.

Use Your Subconscious

"I can go to bed with a problem, sleep, and my brain works out a solution!"

—Selina Danielle, UK

I'm like Selina in this way: my subconscious can really help me out.

Here's a small example:

I love sleeping on my side, but I want to sleep on my back at least some of the night, too, because it's better for my neck. **But I've never been able** *to fall asleep* **on my back.**

Then I somehow got the idea to whisper to my subconscious mind before sleep, that I wanted to sleep on my back in the night, and it worked!

I do it every night now, and it works every night. I make sure I open my eyes when I whisper my request to myself, just to really get my own attention and make an impression on myself, so I'll remember. I'll say: "Joni, turn onto your back in the night."

Then, I wake up on my back. (Also good for smoothing lines on the face. LOL.)

Now I've begun to tell myself other things I want to wake up with: gratitude to be alive; a relaxed nervous system; a hopeful attitude; a healthy body filled with light.

There are lots of inspiring thinkers out there who believe that our subconscious mind hears what our conscious mind says about itself, and makes those things happen.

Prayers before sleep: makes sense.

Affirmations/Self Talk

I love affirmations! Just love them. If I'm in a hard place and I create or find the exactly right sentence, and start saying it to myself, I can at least begin to lift myself out of my low self-esteem, paralyzing inaction, or some other crap mindset I'm in.

According to the classic book *The Power of Your Subconscious Mind*, by Joseph Murphy, the subconscious mind does the bidding of the conscious mind.

The subconscious isn't concerned with good or bad: It simply takes orders and tries to bring about events to support what the conscious mind says.

And the problem is that the conscious mind is never silent and we don't choose the majority of our thoughts. The mind picks them up from our experiences and environment—memories, people, TV, social media, magazine photos—the list goes on.

And so many of our thoughts are negative: My hair's horrible; I just can't do that; It's one f*cking thing after another; He's such an idiot; She never listens; I just can't pay attention; I'm not ready for that!

If we go around letting these negative thoughts run free, they become self-fulfilling prophesies. We convince ourselves they're true and they become true.

So, creating positive statements to repeat throughout your days can counteract negative thoughts and expectations, and create a supportive scaffolding for your mind and your life.

But don't fake an affirmation! In other words, don't say something so far from your reality that you can't really believe it. Instead, spend time fashioning your thoughts into a positive statement that you can actually believe.

In other words, if you're heavily in debt, don't create an over-the-top affirmation like "I'm a debt-free millionaire!" because you probably can't believe that at that point. And affirmations work when you can say them with emotion and excitement.

So if you don't believe in a particular affirmation, it'll be useless.

But if you put some real effort into creating a great affirmation, you can come up with a very positive statement that excites you.

Suppose, instead of saying "I'm a debt-free millionaire!," you said, "I have everything I need to become financially secure?"

See the difference? To me, the second one feels really good. I can get behind that with energy—and get energy from it!

Once you settle on a great affirmation, write it on a note somewhere on your phone, computer, or a piece of paper and keep glancing at it throughout the day until you've memorized it.

Then stick with that one, single statement for at least a week—maybe a month—and repeat it throughout the day. After saying it to yourself for a while, it will begin to take on a life of its own.

You'll see: it'll start popping into your head throughout the day. And it will feed your motivation to do what it is you want to do.

You can also shout your affirmation if you're alone somewhere (like a car). This might make you feel like a nut, but I think it's a powerful form of healing and I admire people who do it (including myself).

Groundhog Day with a Difference

I've been using another powerful exercise that is helping me actualize the changes I want to make in my life—whatever they are that day or week. It builds on the previous two entries, Using Your Subconscious and Affirmations/Self Talk.

And the easy thing about this exercise is that you don't have to decide what to work on: The exercise itself immediately shows you what to work on. Let me explain.

It's best to do the exercise before bed (but you could do it anytime).

Let's say it's the end of the day and you're in bed.

You close your eyes, quiet down, and start remembering what happened that day: **You review your day.**

And when you come upon something that didn't feel good, or you wished had gone differently, you stop there. And you begin using your (amazing ADHD) imagination by picturing the event having gone the way you *wish it had gone.*

That's right: You use your imagination to "revise" the event by imagining it all having gone really well. **You become a filmmaker and you envision a whole little scene.**

Say I'm doing this—reviewing my day—and remember how burdened I felt that I never called back my friend—I'll call her Claire—after having promised that I would.

I feel really crummy about myself that I've promised I'd call her more than once, and haven't, and now I've done it again.

So I set the facts of what I've done (or neglected to do) aside, and start picturing calling her on my phone.

I make it as vivid as I can: I picture myself sitting in my favorite spot and picking up my phone. I check contacts in my phone app, pull up her name, and hit "call." I hear it ring. And then Claire—(I love her!)—answers. And I say, "How are you sweetie?" And I imagine her voice saying that she's good and she's so glad to hear from me.

Doing this in my imagination makes it easier to do it in real life the next time.

Create Slogans

Riffing off my previous entry about the transformative value of using affirmations, I also use slogans to stay on track.

A slogan is a short affirmative statement that is easy to remember. It can even be well-known. "Easy does it," comes to mind as one. Or, "You can do this," or "God heals," or "One step at a time," or "I'm not alone," or "We can do hard things," or "I love you, Joni."

Seasonal Affective Disorder Lamps (Let the Light Shine)

I live in a small town near Boston. Believe me, I fantasize about California or somewhere warmer all the time. But this is where I live, and I have to love what I have, so I do.

But this sun setting around 4 p.m. shite? Yikes, not so good. It's Dec. 14 now, and my phone says that sunset will be at 4:11 p.m. Can you believe it?

It's so funny what all of us New Englanders say to comfort ourselves and each other all fall: "In one more week, on Dec. 21, it'll be the winter solstice, the shortest daylight day of the year. And the next day, on Dec. 22, daylight time will start to grow longer!"

But meanwhile, the lack of light is implicated in increased depression or sadness in people. And I see that this is true for me. So I've been using full-spectrum, natural light lamps, aka seasonal affective disorder (SAD) lamps, for several years to brighten the room I'm in—and my spirits.

There are guidelines about how much exposure you're supposed to get when using one of these lamps to help reverse the effects of low light. (These guidelines have to do with the strength of the particular lamp and your distance from it.) I'm not sure what those are—you have to look them up—but I find that just having a bright, sunshiny light on the table next to me lifts my spirits. It has to do with how we get energy from sunlight, via our retinas, and how that regulates hormones, like **serotonin**, and more.

Plants aren't the only living forms that rely on the sun. Get a lamp if you can. They get me through the winter.

Control Screen Time

I've long known about creating healthy boundaries in relationships with others. But it's new to me to realize **that I've got some seriously deficient boundaries around using the Internet.** It's the biggest intruder into my life and mind these days.

Our brains need time to do nothing in order to function best. **Artists aren't the only ones who are creative**—that's a misuse of words. **All people are creative all the time. And our minds create the most and the best stuff when our brains are free to be idle for periods of awake time.**

But modern life is really screwing with us. I know you know this, but most of us are spending very little, if any, time just being: standing and waiting, sitting and looking, walking quietly, whatever. We're on our devices.

You see it everywhere: Otherwise reasonable, interesting, good, fun people are standing in line waiting for coffee, scrolling the screens of their phones! We're addicted to the excitement and stimulation of a quick hit of something online. And the irony is that most of what we're scrolling for on our devices isn't important or even that interesting to us.

The addiction is to the instantaneous action of moving from site to site, or comment to comment. Lightning f a s t! Although the web and ADHD are a match made in heaven,

ADHDers aren't the only ones affected. **Dr. Edward Hallowell** believes the continuous eruption of information that bombards us has created a condition in the general public that closely resembles ADHD.

Minutes and hours lost to scrolling Facebook, Twitter, Pinterest, Instagram, TikTok, Apple News, online window shopping and more are taking a massive toll on us.

Do you think you could or should impose some boundaries around your Internet use?

Every day, people join the movement to unplug (in various ways).

Can you not use your devices for an hour?

One Formula for Making a Change

I like this guy who's written a few extremely simple books on ADHD and has a blog. He's a psychiatrist who learned he had ADHD in his 60s. His name is Doug Puryear.

He works a lot with strategies. And **his formula** for making changes to help with things that mess him up is the following:

1. Identify a problem;
2. Make a strategy;
3. Make the strategy a rule;
4. Make the rule a habit.

Here's an example of what he means:

I notice that lately I've been getting really side-tracked by random thoughts that send me off on tangents researching or window shopping (online) when I'm working. I would really like to find a solution to this problem to at least diminish how often it happens.

Okay, so I've identified the problem. (Going off on tangents researching or otherwise pursuing something online that pops into my mind.)

The strategy I've decided on to remedy this problem is to jot down on paper what it is I want to go racing after. Writing it down helps relieve my impulse to go pursue whatever it is that's tempting me and resist racing off after it.

Since I always have my notebook with me, I jot it down there. With the date. (I add the date to make it more substantial.)

After I jot it down, I feel relieved of it being on my mind so I know it's a good strategy.

After doing it a few times, I decide to make it a rule, which means I'm going to make a big effort to stick with this strategy.

So when a thought comes up to go look for something online that I suddenly think I must research, I recognize the problem, and remember that I have a strategy. And, if I keep sticking with my chosen strategy over and over again, it becomes a habit.

Voila!

Frozen Vegetables: Seriously

If you suffer from what-the-flying-f*ck-am-I-going-to-make-for-dinner … or … torture yourself wanting to get more vegetables into your diet but keep finding them rotted in the fridge, I've got a trick for you.

Frozen string beans. I'm telling you. They're as good as fresh green beans you buy at the grocery store except for maybe when they're in season. I get them at both Whole Foods and Trader Joe's. You bring an inch of water to a boil and pour the whole bag in, cover it, and bring it back up to the boil. And drain.

Frozen corn is great, too. I mean, what's not to love about corn? (But I think green veggies have more nutrients.)

Get Dressed First Thing in the Morning

If you have a job and have to be out the door early, getting dressed first thing is a given. But if you work at home, you might not, yet I'm willing to bet you'd have a better day if you did.

I've always been a freelancer. I work at home mostly. And in the dead of winter (and the dead of Covid), it's very tempting to not change out of my pajamas. But when I get up, wash my face, put my hair up, put a little makeup on and some real clothes, it signals my brain that I'm open for business.

And I am! Being dressed makes it easier to do the next right thing because I don't have to go get dressed first. I already am dressed.

Being dressed puts me one step closer to getting things done.

Being dressed changes my mindset and signals me that I'm ready to start working at my desk. Getting dressed makes me more productive.

Not only am I ready—if someone knocks on the door or I really need to do an errand out in the world—but it makes me feel better about myself.

Getting dressed lifts my mood. It makes me feel more a part of the world, more confident, more motivated. And when I'm in a better mood, I'm better to everyone I encounter.

Getting dressed helps define the day from the night.

Some people say getting dressed is part of good mental hygiene. How's that for you? Good mental hygiene: Good term!

Make Your Bed

I'm not a f*cking drill sergeant. You can't bounce a dime off my bed. But I have, in the past year, been making my bed as soon as I get up.

I gotta say, doing it almost kills me. I want to get to that cup of coffee f a s t. But I've been doing it for a year now, and I really like how it makes me feel.

It's so helpful because it sends me off into my day feeling like I've already accomplished something.

It also makes me feel happy to know that come night, I have a nice bed waiting for me. It's like a period at the end of a sentence: It wraps up the night and readies me for the day.

Sit on the Floor for a Minute

This is a pretty eccentric suggestion, but I can't help it: Sit on the floor.

I'm not kidding. I mean it.

There's something very grounding about sitting on the floor (LOL).

It can be a small practice in and of itself.

First, you have to find a position that's comfortable.

Maybe you're flexible enough to do it easily and can sit cross-legged, or atop your folded legs, accordion style, no problem.

But plenty of people can't sit on the floor and never do. (My husband can't really—not comfortably enough to stay for ten minutes. He can run for an hour playing soccer, but he isn't flexible like that.)

If you make it a little practice to sit on the floor, you'll get more agile as time goes on, and stronger.

For me, I want to be able to sit on the floor comfortably until the day I die. It's a big thing to me. I really cherish being able to sit on the floor comfortably.

And, meanwhile, while you're down there on the floor, *take a minute.*

There's something so wonderfully calming about sitting on the floor.

Don't take your f*cking phone out. Just sit there.

Take a breath.

Close your eyes, if you want to, and feel into yourself sitting there.

Even only one (whole) minute is good.

Consider Yoga

Considering that impulsivity, anxiety, and restlessness are big issues for me, I'm all for anything that can calm me down.

Yoga classes do that for me. So much.

I know there's a bit of a backlash against yoga: that it's so trendy, or that people seem superior about doing it—holier than thou, maybe. But I can tell you that I've done yoga for a long time and **for me it's been the one activity (especially when done in a class with others and a good, lovely teacher) that makes me quiet down almost completely.**

If you've been wanting to try a yoga class but haven't taken the plunge because you can't get a grip on which class to take, below is a description of the nine most popular classes.

All About the Different Yoga Classes

Note: For your first class, if possible, find one that's recommended for beginners.

Hatha

Hatha is a general term for the physical practice of doing yoga poses (postures/asanas). At most good yoga studios, a Hatha class will be a good introductory class for newcomers. The instructor will demonstrate the pose while describing how to do it and then talk you back out of the pose and into the next one. Hatha is also beneficial for more experienced students. While a beginner will be learning the positioning and alignment of a pose, an experienced student can take the same pose further toward its full expression. And both will be doing yoga and reaping its benefits.

Iyengar

Iyengar is a yoga style that emphasizes extremely precise alignment in poses. It is excellent for beginners because correct alignment in poses is what makes the pose work for you and optimizes its benefits. Alignment means that you learn which parts of your body—in a particular pose—are stretching, or contracting, or lifted, or twisting, or rotating inward or outward. All these actions happen at the same time, using different parts of your body, in a single pose. Iyengar gives you a solid foundation that will serve you in other types of classes where the poses flow swiftly into one another.

Vinyasa or Flow

Vinyasa Flow-style yoga classes are based on moving from one pose to another in a flowing action, with a special emphasis on synchronizing your breath with your movement. Generally, when you do a movement that contracts your body in on itself (like bending forward), you exhale, and when you lift or arch your spine in a back-bendy, expansive direction, you inhale. Flow sequences can be long. Or they can be as short and simple as the popular warm-up flow called Cat-Cow. You start Cat-Cow on all fours (aka tabletop). You then alternate between arching your back and looking upward, like a cow, and contracting your back, like an angry cat, while inhaling and exhaling, respectively.

Power Yoga

These classes are fast-moving Vinyasa Flow classes that are often performed in heated rooms. They are good for very fit people *who have already mastered the alignment of the basic poses in Hatha or Iyengar classes*, so that when they fly from pose to pose, they're maintaining the proper alignment of the postures.

Hot Yoga

Hot yoga is generally the same as Power Yoga, but it's always done in a room that's heated to at least 95 degrees and humidified by hot steam! (I can't handle it—I get too hot.)

Ashtanga

These yoga classes follow a strict series of the same poses performed sequentially in a fast-moving, strenuous Vinyasa Flow with synchronized breath. Ashtanga has a primary, intermediate, and advanced series. Ashtanga is extremely strenuous and is good for those who have developed a very strong foundation in yoga and are extremely fit. Hot and Power yoga take much of their style from Ashtanga.

Yin Yoga

In Yin Yoga, poses are held for several minutes at a time, and the goal is to melt (release/relax) into the pose—right at the edge of comfort and discomfort. Yin Yoga increases flexibility, steadies the mind, and loosens fascia—the overlooked connective tissue that surrounds and supports all parts of our bodies. A Yin class should be okay for a beginner, but always make sure to tell the teacher that you're new.

Kundalini

Kundalini Yoga classes consist of movements that are mostly different from the regular canon of basic yoga poses you'll see in all the other types of yoga classes. Kundalini combines chanting, breathing, and doing specific sets of movements, known as kriyas. I don't recommend Kundalini as a good class for a beginner interested in yoga because what you'll learn won't be directly applicable to all the other styles of yoga. Still, if you're curious, try a class. You may love it.

I highly recommend starting with a beginner Hatha or Iyengar class, if you can find one. But whichever class you take, be sure to tell the instructor, before class, that you're just starting out.

Getting detailed instruction in the fundamental poses will set you up with a strong, solid foundation that will serve you well in any type of yoga class you take.

Fidgeting Can Help

I love watching my sister Toni's foot when we're sitting around.

She'll often be moving it up and down, the way people do. **To me, it's almost like she's purring. It not only soothes her, it soothes me.**

Experts say that **fidgeting**—mindless movement a person can do while doing something else—**helps us stay focused by giving our restless brains something to do!**

I had a therapist who suggested I get a special object, like a stone, to carry around and rub. That had the added benefit of acting like a touchstone: I could go touch it and remember that I wanted to take a long breath in and out whenever I touched it.

Remember worry beans? I like those.

I was always a big doodler in school.

There are all kinds of fidget tools out there or you can make your own.

Exercise for Short Bursts Throughout the Day

According to brain experts, physical exercise causes the body and brain to produce a bunch of feel-good chemicals including our motivating friends—**dopamine**, and other neurotransmitters, including superstars **serotonin**, **epinephrine**, and **norepinephrine**.

Even a minute or two-minute burst of exercise will activate these sensitive compounds and a range of others that nourish, housekeep, and invigorate brain cells.

Which is so great—and good and useful—because for one thing, it's so much easier to get myself to do a minute of exercise than a longer session.

It takes me a whole lot less motivation to sidle up to the exercise bike, sit on the seat, and pedal for a minute.

And once I've gone for a minute, I might want to do a second minute. (You start to feel good from the first minute, which fuels wanting to do a second!)

If you're at work someplace, you can probably find a way to get in a couple minutes of exercise—going up flights of stairs a couple times, or walking somewhere, back and forth.

Make these two-minute exercise breaks a constant part of your life, and you'd be doing a really good thing for your body and mind.

Be Your Own Friend

"The core and the surface are essentially the same ..."

—Lao Tzu

If you're in a bad place, you could try and break the cycle by smiling.

I'm not suggesting you do this at times when you need to be present to sadness or pain. **I'm not suggesting that you deny your painful feelings.**

But I am suggesting that at certain times when you're irritated, feeling blah, or at a loss about what your next move should be, smiling could help.

Lifting the corners of your mouth upward sends signals to some part of our mind-body that actually shifts hormones and other chemicals and perks us up! At times, *faking it until you make it* gets you where you'd like to go.

Instead of smiling, you might do a jaunty walk. Or blast some music and dance. Be playful.

I remember my godchild Lily putting on a Halloween costume on Halloween one year when she was staying home alone. I thought that was so cool. I liked that a lot!

We're the only ones in our own heads: Why not tend them like a loving gardener or the general manager of a five-star hotel rather than a derelict apartment complex?

Begin Again

Come, come wherever you are.
Wanderer, worshiper, lover of leaving.
It doesn't matter!
Ours is not a caravan of despair.
Come, even if you have broken your vows
A thousand times
Come! Yet again! Come, come!

—Rumi

If you have ADHD, things will be easier if you can accept that you're often going to have to start some things again: that you're going to have to do a lot of coming back to something you dropped and pick it back up.

If you can, just start whatever it is you want, again.

Think of this as the cost of doing business.

You may have wanted to do something at an earlier time and quit, and then find yourself wanting to do it again. And maybe you take another hiatus from it, then two months later you're wanting to do it again.

I say, just start again. If this is the row you have to hoe to get where you want to go, then do it.

Just start again and f*ck those negative thoughts that criticize you for your process. It's what it is!

And, yes, it is a pain, but there's a lot of pain in life.

This is okay. You can start again. It's good. You're doing what you have to do for yourself. You're working with your type of brain. Good!

Tiny Sensory Sensitivity Hack When Shopping

"I get sensory overload in restaurants where people are drinking, music, chitter-chatter, noisy children, coffee machine, glasses clanging, cutlery being put into a tray, etc. I cannot focus on someone two feet away from my face but can catch a conversation 15 meters away."

—Selina Danielle, UK

I sometimes get overloaded in restaurants, too, like Selina, especially if their menus are big. And my overload isn't confined to restaurants, but can happen in any environment where a lot of things are going on.

Some days my brain is more energetic than other days.

If I'm not feeling my best, and have to go into a big store, I'll walk around quietly looking at the floor as I cruise the aisles so my eyes don't expose my brain to the thousands of items in its purview every second.

It's no big deal, no one notices, but it gives my brain a little break.

Suiting Up and Showing Up

They say it in 12-Step programs: suit up and show up. I find this slogan super helpful sometimes when I'm really dragging and dreading doing something.

Sometimes it's impossible or impractical to untangle all the reasons why I'm resistant to doing a particular thing, on a particular day, and it's better to just do it even though it feels unsettled.

There are so many things that can contribute to not wanting to do something you've said you'd do.

You could be **worried** about having to talk about an issue you're undecided on. Or you **don't have anything to wear**; your **hair looks awful**; you don't want to risk the chance that **you might end up embarrassed about something you do or say that will leave you in a prolonged stew of painful self-criticism: rejected, dejected, and hurt.** Or **you haven't made any food to take,** gotten a gift, or feel like you **can't spend the money** involved.

But no matter what comprises your particular resistance, *sometimes* it works to just screw all that stuff and **simply suit up and show up.**

This means that sometimes you don't have to figure everything out. You just sidestep all your internal BS and do the thing.

God Box

Many people assume that if someone says they believe in God that they're saying they believe in a bearded humanoid figure in the sky that controls everything that happens. And a heaven above and a burning hell below. I don't believe those things.

But I absolutely believe in God—and I also believe that I can't know exactly what God is.

Still, I have faith that God is a power for good that I can access within myself.

I could talk forever about my beliefs and experiences of my "God," but **all I want to tell you about here is my God Box and suggest that you use one.**

So, what it is, is a small wooden box that lives in one of my bureau drawers. Someone I love—Nina—gave it to me. And inside it are small pieces of paper folded up, private-like. And written on each piece of paper is something I want God to handle for me. Like fear of losing a job; sadness at someone's sickness; grief over a loss; regret. And on and on.

The idea is to surrender your struggles, fears, and burdens to some power bigger than yourself.

When I go look inside my God Box months later, I see that many of the things I've put in it have been resolved.

It's a relief just writing something down and putting it in the box. It's as though I'm asking another part of myself to carry the weight of the difficult emotion I'm struggling with.

I believe that we humans are much more than we appear to be: that we're not just bodies and minds that can be measured and known. I believe that a bigger part of us exists in another dimension or realm of being beyond conscious thought, although I don't know what it is. I think that life might be a dream that a bigger part of me is dreaming. Something like that.

Anyway. Make yourself a God Box if you can remotely get behind the idea. They're so sweet.

PART IV E

Feelings

Breaking Through Discouragement—and Addiction

Sometimes just naming a thing that's bothering you helps make it stop bothering you.

I recognized a while ago that I can get discouraged pretty easily when slogging through something I'm trying to do.

It's a thing: discouragement. It says, "You can't do this! This isn't for you! Forget about it!"

At times like that, years ago, I used to take a hit of cannabis and suddenly a voice in my head would say, "Honey, of course you can do this. Just stick with it. You were born for this. Don't give up!"

That worked very nicely—for a couple hours. Getting high really did help me see that my negative thoughts weren't the truth.

The problem was, though, that once high, I couldn't muster the personal power to do all I had to do to be part of the world. Not only that, but I became highly addicted to cannabis. Most people don't think that is possible, but I promise you, it is. I can't stop using it once I start. The only way for me to have any freedom is total abstinence.

Sadly, ADHDers' have a much higher than average incidence of addiction of any sort—alcohol absolutely included. I can tell you that addiction is a dead end and that the only way through it is abstinence. And that *you can get through it*. Nobody could love cannabis more than I do, and if I can do it, you can too. **(If you need some support with this, feel free to get in touch with me.)**

Meanwhile, without dope, I've learned other ways to gentle myself through periods of discouragement.

If you're feeling discouraged today—thinking you can't do what you're wanting to do—take a moment and give yourself a nice talking to.

"You can do it, sweetie," you might say. Or "you can do it, Dude! Just stick with it!"

Then take a break if you need to. Call someone and tell them you're discouraged. Reach out to someone and connect any way you can. Maybe read this again or go to a cafe and look the counter person in the eye, ask how they're doing, and really listen to what they say.

There are so many ways to disrupt a counterproductive energy flow like discouragement, so suit up and go do one of them.

I'm holding the space for you. Go grab it!

About Anxiety

"The minute I think about having to focus on something or complete a task that requires my focus, I get anxious. First, I have to calm the anxieties that surge up. This is the war I have. Me vs. anxiety. **If I can send anxiety retreating, then I have a chance to block distractions.** *My war against anxiety requires medication, my dogs, lots of rest, good friends and family, and fun. Hair twirling, too. LOL.*

Writing with **pen and paper helps me***. Something about the hand and brain connection works for me. Plus there are no distracting apps or search bars when* **writing longhand***! A dog in my lap is a must for when I get anxious or distracted. I pat and enjoy him then get calmed and go back to my task.* **Music helps** *as well. It's always been a stress-buster for me.* **Singing out loud** *on occasion helps as well. It gets excess energy out, as does* **moving/bouncing my legs***. If I don't get rid of excess energy, it makes it that much harder to focus.*

—Mandy, a school administrator

All of this is just to say that whatever's good for generalized anxiety disorders can be useful for ADHD. Namely, calming down however you can. The next three entries are some things I do to calm my anxiety.

Also, if you're implementing any strategies that lessen your various troublesome traits—procrastination, impulsivity, indecision, shame, forgetfulness—they're likely lowering your general level of anxiety, too.

(There's more than one way to skin a cat. Right?) (Ouch: the poor cat!)

Breathing

It almost always irritates me when somebody tells me to take a breath (go f*ck yourself I think.) (FYI, that curse makes me laugh and I use it a lot with affection and humor.)

Yet every time I close my eyes—at a red light, standing in a line, sitting with a cup of something—if I just take a long deep breath in and then out, I feel calmer.

Breathing is extremely trippy if you ponder it. Isn't it? There's a lot of science around the tremendous benefits of breathing exercises.

I actually have to hand it to myself for once: I have a pretty good intentional breathing practice that I learned years ago in one yoga class. It's one of the treasures of my life.

You think it isn't going to do anything, but if you can stop and take a deep breath, or two deep breaths, or several, or five minutes' worth, it's highly likely that you'll calm down at least some.

I understand that at times you won't be able to make yourself do it. But, when you can, give it a try.

Dealing with Anger

We know that many women with ADHD have strong positive and negative emotions and a hard time regulating them. A fast, hot rage is one of my most damaging ones.

And when it happens, the first thing I try hard to do is hold my tongue.

I do this to stop myself from lashing out because **if I say something cutting or mean, it ends up making me feel ten times worse afterward.**

I am in no way suggesting that you stifle your anger. (I'm totally in favor of expressing dark feelings—in safe environments—so they can evolve and move on.)

But I am suggesting that a first step **at working on erupting rage is to attempt to bypass saying or doing something mean that would just dig you deeper into a negative spiral.**

So the second the rage hits, I have to start working on ways to control my initial response.

This is hard. I'll be in a state like the Hulk—really angry! And that anger wants the release of telling the person how angry I am and letting them know that I think their behavior is awful: I want to hurt them.

Often, I have to remove myself from the environment in order to calm down, so I don't lash out. I might go outside, if possible, or into the bathroom if there's nowhere else to be alone.

Depending on the situation, I might write about how angry I am. Or call a good friend who knows how this can happen to me. Or I give myself a good talking-to, reminding myself that I'm more than my anger. That I know it hurts. That I will take care of the perceived injustice, but that I need to calm down first. I tell myself I love myself and that I'm going to be okay.

Once I've reined my rage back in, I can decide whether to talk to the person about the issue that made me so mad. But I've got to be in control of what I say to do this, otherwise it's best to put off conversing.

One of the hardest parts about getting enraged is that if I don't handle myself skillfully, I end up getting depressed for a day or two.

Over the years, and with therapy and a modicum of self-caring techniques and awareness at play, I've gotten a lot better.

I've come to understand that becoming flooded with rage involves a disconnection from the authentic, adult self in me. I lose touch with the rest of my life experience and only have access to the rage. An emotionally skilled person, or an otherwise less highly strung one, is often able to navigate anger and arguments without getting flooded.

The less time I spend in rage, blame, hurt, and other hard places, the quicker I can get back my equilibrium. And the first step for me is holding my tongue.

Courage

It takes courage just to be human.

I watched Pete Buttigieg yesterday (it's September 2019) announce his candidacy for president at his first nationally televised rally and was deeply moved and inspired by his courage.

One of the camera angles was shot in profile, showing him just standing there listening to the crowd cheer him.

And you could see that he was standing with his arms just hanging down: a vulnerable stance. (On stage, or anywhere before a crowd, it's so much safer-feeling to lean on a podium or have your arms gesturing like they do when speaking.)

Life requires great courage. If nothing else, courage.

What would be brave of me today?

I'd like to be free of shame like Pete Buttigieg, who has the courage to be honest and *open about a part of himself that society still stigmatizes massively.*

I'm thinking he's one emotionally healthy guy to have his head on that straight.

I hope you can be brave today.

Forgiveness

I recently wrote the following entry about forgiveness and then came across an essay by a woman who lost her leg in a car accident and learned to forgive the driver of the other car who caused the crash.

Although I believe that everything I've written below is true, my words feel presumptuous or inadequate for anyone whose anger was caused by someone who hurt them as badly as this woman was hurt.

I was going to throw out this entry after reading the aforementioned essay, then decided to keep it in. But if you've been badly hurt, please forgive me for approaching forgiveness in such a light way.

These words are helpful to me with everyday angers and resentments—dozens of which are always springing up.

—JW

Imagine if some galactic dust blew across the Earth one day causing every grievance in the heads and hearts of every person on Earth to disappear instantaneously. Every war would end!

But that's almost impossible to *even imagine*: **The world seems to be held together with blame and anger. Our hatreds and** resentments, invisible though they may be, are stronger than steel.

It's mind-blowing to realize that what binds us in constant battle starts inside our own heads.

You'd think we could just change our minds. Just give up the fight.

I want this: I want to give up the fight: **to release resentment and anger the minute they arise.** I think of it as **personal disarmament**.

But it is not easy to let go of *righteous* anger and blame and forgive the other guy, especially when I don't condone, accept, or agree with what they've done that I **resent**.

Still, I want to forgive them because it makes me feel badly to hang on to anger. I don't want it. I don't want to be attached to the object of my anger through the heavy energy of my own negative feelings. I want to be released from the whole thing.

Holding onto resentment, blame, and anger only hurts me! I feel like shit when I'm resentful toward someone or something.

There are so many benefits to forgiving another person. Forgiveness is actually so deeply important, so far-reaching, so sacred a dynamic that I'm not sure I can do it any justice with these few thoughts.

To clarify: I'm not saying that forgiving someone or something means that I accept, agree, or condone the thing I'm forgiving.

But I've learned that forgiving others allows me to forgive myself for all the things I've imagined I've done wrong. Forgiving someone else sets *me* free.

One way I've learned to forgive someone is to take a moment every day for two weeks and wish good things for them. Use your imagination to picture the person doing well at something or having something wonderful happen to them.

I don't find this easy: A part of me does not want to do it. But when I do—the few times I've really done this—it's worked. A little time will have passed after the two weeks, and I'll be reminded of what that person did that I was so angry about, and I won't feel anything much. The charge will have been neutralized.

If you pray, you can pray that your Higher Self, Higher Power, the Universe, or your God remove your anger. You can explain that you know that your anger is only hurting you and you don't want it anymore.

Or do like some Shamans and talk to your anger and thank it for helping protect you back when you encountered the hurt that angered you. And then tell it that you no longer need its protection and want to move on to other feelings.

Can you forgive someone for something? Do you wish you could? Might you try?

One Way to Get Around Emotional Dysregulation: Do You Want to be Happy, or Right?

A lot of women with ADHD have strong emotional reactions to people, places, and things. I found myself having one of those yesterday. Here's what happened.

My husband and I were in the car. And we started talking about a certain problem issue that I won't get into here. And he started saying this thing about the issue that he's said before. And it irritated me—a lot—because he'd said the same thing several times before, and I didn't see how it could help us explore the issue further toward a solution.

And I got really annoyed and started criticizing him for always saying the same thing, and I became, zero to sixty, mean to him.

And right then, *right then,* **I remembered that I do not want to be this way.** I do not want to be critical of him and unkind. And not only that, but his input was probably important and all I was doing was shutting him down from explaining it more.

You could say that I had a flash of enlightenment and saw that there was absolutely no reason at all for me to get all critical. I saw that I was being manipulated by some ego desire to be superior and contrary. That my criticism was an ugly way to be and not at all in keeping with my values: I want to be kind to people and focus on the love that is the ground of our shared being.

And I remembered what my yoga teacher says: to have kind thoughts and say kind words. And I remembered, too, Ram Dass's lifelong effort to be with people as souls, not as egos. And I remembered that question I've heard a lot: Do you want to be right, or happy? **And I knew one hundred percent that I want to be kind, happy, and *with* another person, not against them.**

So I dropped my criticism like a hot potato. I told him I was sorry and asked him some questions about this piece of the situation that so interested him.

And I learned something.

Off Days: Out Sick with ADHD (Take a Mental Health Day)

One of the most damning results of our culture's general ignorance about the effects of various neurodiversities is the absence of almost any societal recognition that people can be having a bad mental/emotional health day!

It's totally cool if you're out sick with a flu, a bad back, a urinary tract infection, or a torn meniscus.

But what about if you're feeling especially overwhelmed, depressed, foggy-headed, or too sensitive to handle the world at large?

I'll tell you what happens to a lot of us: We lie.

Instead of being truthful, we feel we have to lie.

I have an acquaintance and I know she does this: She feels too humiliated to say that she's not mentally and emotionally up for going out that day. And you can't blame her: Society certainly doesn't model any recognition of the need to take time off to get well when you're hurting in some inner, invisible way.

This is such a glaring lack in our health care ethic and culture that it's hard to believe: Here we are in the midst of an opioid epidemic—along with widespread teenage depression, anxiety, and suicide—and yet we, as a society, don't generally acknowledge mental/emotional illnesses, disorders, and neurodiversities!

To be fair: Some workplaces allow you to say that you're taking a mental health day, so at least that's a start.

This needs to change because lying about, and hiding, how you're feeling enforces a sense of shame about neurodiversity. **Lying like this is a terrible abandonment of the self.** Nobody should have to do that.

When I can't make a date of any sort, I've learned to simply say, "I'm so sorry but I'm just not feeling up to it today."

Bathrooms as Sanctuaries

Ha! If you need a minute—when you're out somewhere—remember you can always go to a bathroom where you can have a few minutes in a low-stimulus space and gather yourself.

I've been known to get down on my knees and pray in more than one bathroom. (I understand that this conjures the specter of germs, etc., but some bathrooms are nice and clean and I'm not a germaphobe anyway. Whatever: I've done it.) And you don't have to get on your knees to pray: It's just an outward stance that cues us, internally, that we're placing ourselves before a spiritual power.

In any case, you don't even have to pray! You can just take a few moments to calm yourself down. Check on any notes you may have brought with you—**peoples' names, questions you have, ideas you want to contribute.** You can **review** any **affirmations** you're working with and your **intentions** for the event: **to remember that you are safe**; to remember **that you don't have to prove your worth**; to remember **that you don't need anyone's approval**; to remember **that you're part of it all**; to **remember that people aren't focused on you anyway—but are most likely thinking about, and being inside of, their own experience.**

I remember being at this dance party in eighth grade in my friend's basement, and people were making out and I didn't want to. I went upstairs and went into the bathroom and felt so safe in there. I don't remember what happened after that—I think I asked to call my parents to pick me up—but I always remember the relief of closing and locking the bathroom door behind me. Whew! (P.S. I've since more than made up for my early revulsion to making out.)

PART IV F

Relationships

The Pause Button

Once I was at a party talking to a really fascinating woman. I'm quite sure she has ADHD. It was at the end of the night and most people were leaving, but she and I were still talking our heads off.

And then the coolest thing happened. **Her husband pulled out a white business card and handed it to her. All it said, in tiny black letters, was "Stop talking now."**

I loved the guy for that. He was interrupting her impulsive excitement and reminding her of what they'd obviously agreed upon prior to that evening: that she sometimes needed help remembering not to talk so much.

This is similar to what I do to control my impulsivity. It isn't rocket science, but it isn't easy. And I have to do it all myself, whereas he was helping her.

The first step is to develop enough self-awareness to recognize that I'm about to do something that's just popped into my head or that I'm on a tear.

Often, it's me impulsively offering something I later won't want to, or can't, actually deliver. Or interrupting people, talking way too much, or buying something.

You have to make it a priority to gain enough self-awareness to recognize impulsivity triggers and urges when they come up. Journaling that this is your intention will help. Writing some external cues about it on a Post-it note, like "watch yourself, Joan!" helps, too.

You can also review past situations where you've been regrettably impulsive and figure out if a particular mood triggered you. For me, it's often excitement. For some people, it's loneliness or some other low feeling. **Once you've identified your mood triggers you can be especially vigilant when they hit.**

If you've become pretty good at recognizing an urge to do something impulsively, you can find a way to pause before you do it.

When the awareness hits, you could say the word "pause!" or "breathe," and actually take a deep breath. You could wear an **elastic band** and snap it. You could touch a necklace you wear that you've designated to remind you to pause. You could remind yourself before an event or date **that your intention is to pause** before acting on an impulse. If you're on the phone, or even sitting at a cafe with someone, you can have **your little notebook** in your hand and jot down what you want to say so you'll remember it and not have to interrupt. You could **memorize a couple questions to ask yourself,** like "will doing this be **good for me?" or "when I wake up tomorrow, will I want to follow through on this?"**

Maybe you'll discover that some of your impulsivity comes from people-pleasing: that you grew up taking care of other people and think you have to rush in and help everyone. This is a toughie. But if you become accustomed to recognizing impulsivity arising, **you can create that little pause that gives you the time to restrain yourself.**

When you create the time to think before you answer, you can see that you don't always have to go for it. And that if you really want to say whatever it is, or offer whatever it is, you can do it—later.

About Apologizing

I just had a solid lesson in apologizing the other day.

I'd said something to my great friend Jane about a thing she did that bothered me, and I thought the way I'd said it was kind of kiddingly. But the subject came up the next day that my comment had bothered Jane a bit.

And I was going over this with our other great friend, Nathalie, because she'd heard the exchange. And while I was sure my comment was a playful way of saying how I'd been bothered, Nathalie didn't see it that way. She thought my comment was passive aggressive and not so nice. And clearly, since it had bothered Jane, I realized that it hadn't come off as playful.

And although Jane is very loving and wouldn't hold it against me, I wanted to apologize.

So I thought and thought about why I'd said the thing … and what I should say when apologizing.

And I was going over with Nathalie all the ways I could apologize. They all began with "I'm so sorry I hurt your feelings when I said what I said, please forgive me," and then I'd add this or that explanation of my motivations or what I thought hers were when doing the thing that had bothered me.

In other words, I was trying to add on to the apology an alternate way of expressing what had bothered me!

But Nat suggested, "Why don't you just apologize and then see what she says?"

And after going over it a few times, I decided to take her advice: just apologize sincerely but not go on and on about why I thought she'd done what she'd done, or why I'd made the comment I'd made.

All of which would have just complicated the apology.

So I called Jane and apologized really sincerely and stopped speaking.

And Jane came back with the best response, it was so great. And we talked a bit more and it was all very loving and wonderful.

Because I love Jane and Nathalie, this experience made a big impression on me and I think I'll remember it.

I tend to think and talk a lot, but I've learned that I don't have to tell everybody all my complicated inner motivations and what I think theirs are!

I don't have to carry the weight of both sides of a relationship. I only have to keep my side of the street clean.

So this incident cemented in my mind something I'd practiced before, but clearly not well enough: that **it's best and most productive to not complicate an apology, but just apologize, from the heart.**

Do you know what I mean? It was so good!

The Desire to Hit Send

I almost did it the other day: hit "send" on an email to this work acquaintance in which I'd really over-shared. I'm so grateful I didn't send it.

Instead of just apologizing for not having responded to her about a job offer earlier, I wanted to tell her why. And the why had to do with the fact that one of her earlier communiques had hurt my feelings.

So, wanting to be authentic with her, I took great care to write out how I'd been hurt and turned off.

But it was great that I held off on sending the email because I later realized that this woman was not on the same page as I was on this issue: She wouldn't have been able to grasp my in-depth explanation and it would have gummed up the works between us.

Thank God I've had enough experience hitting send too quickly and later regretting it to pause before I sent this one!

The desire to send can be so strong. It's that impulsive urge again: A desire that just wants to do it **now**.

As a general rule, just do not hit send on emails or texts the second you finish writing them. Learn to hold off for a minute.

Stop People Pleasing

Being in agreement with another person is a wonderful, life-affirming experience. The backbone of my happiness is being with people who hold similar world views.

Still, even the closest friends will inevitably have different opinions on some subjects. This is universally true, so **among our basic life skills has to be the ability to express our opinions—without taking or giving offense.**

Growing up, I didn't learn how to be at ease with another person's differing views very well. If my father was in a dark mood and anybody disagreed with him, or doubted his position on something, he exploded. It was terrifying, painful, and damaging.

Meanwhile, I never fully learned that it was totally natural for people to disagree nicely, and not a reason to attack each other or take offense.

And, because I never learned how to express my opinions nicely—and also hated confrontation—I developed the coping mechanism of people-pleasing.

I know I'm not alone. **Many women with ADHD learn to please people and agree with others to avoid being ridiculed for being different:** excitable, enthusiastic, introverted and dreamy, interested in unusual things, unorganized, talkative, inconsistent, lost in thought ... whatever.

So we essentially lied, or lied by omission, and agreed when we did not agree.

But the problem is that it hurts our wholeness (integrity) to conceal our true motives, feelings, and beliefs. To do it is to abandon ourselves.

There is something inherently true and right about being yourself and sharing your particular point of view. Life wants each of us to be our unique selves.

When we hide our true opinions, or simply agree to get by, it takes a toll on us. We feel drained, or out of sorts, or even obsessed with the things we said or didn't say.

Okay, so how to stop people-pleasing? **Here are a few suggestions:**

Stand your ground. It's good and right to say what you feel or believe. You don't have to fight or demand that the other person agree with you. It's natural and okay to have a different opinion on something.

In many situations, it's very useful to simply say, **"Let's agree to disagree."**

It's totally healthy to say no. If asked to do something you don't believe in, say that you're sorry, but it isn't the right thing for you to do. You don't need to justify or lie: Lying to hide your truth will hurt you. If someone is really pushing you, kindly tell them that you understand what they've repeatedly suggested, and that your answer remains the same.

If you don't stand up for yourself, you won't have a self with which to help anyone else in life. And, in my opinion, being of service to others is a great gift.

Asking for Help

"*For it is in giving that we receive,*" says the penultimate line in the widely known St. Francis prayer.

If you don't know the prayer, *it's all about asking to be an instrument of a higher goodness within you.*

I believe that deep down, each of us is hardwired to be good to ourselves and others: to bring love where there is hate, forgiveness where there is injury, etc.

Nobody knows where the prayer came from, but it started showing up in the early 1900s.

I know it might sound very religious to you, but it can also be taken as a non-religious (secular) affirmation to become a better person. A person doesn't have to be a believer in anything but the goodness inherent in her own heart to use this incantation.

All of which is to say that I'm discovering that the line I quoted about giving and receiving is deeply true.

I've always had a hard time asking for some types of help. (Luckily, it's easy for me to ask for help understanding something, or for directions, or as a reporter, for endless clarification on some issue.)

But to ask for help where the other person has to really do something for me? Much harder.

But you know what makes me happiest? When I've been able to help someone else. Bring soup to a neighbor. Call a lonely person. Take a friend to the doctor. Help someone with their computer.

So, giving really is receiving … because when I give, I receive a very good feeling.

Asking for help forms a connection between the receiver and the giver—and connecting with others is one of the most deeply healing, loving things we can do.

Asking for help shows that we're wise enough to be humble: Nobody nowhere knows everything (far from it)!

Asking for some help also lets the other person know that you value their experience.

When you hit a wall, a good way forward is to ask someone for help!

Body Doubling

*"**My parents taught me about partnering with other people to do homework** because we didn't do that growing up—whereas in my kids' school now they actually have team projects.*

But my parents said, 'there's somebody you can study with—find somebody to study with to help you.'

*So that's really what helped me be successful. **My parents got me—they got my strengths, and they got the things I needed to work on.***

It was intuitive on their part. Both my parents are literally all over the place, but they understood themselves. So they were able to take some of the things they learned and give me some of those things. So I was very blessed."

—Yakini, ADHDer, entrepreneur, and mother of two

I do so much better when somebody else even just sits in the same room with me when I'm doing something I'm loath to do, like working on my taxes.

A new-ish theory known as the Orchid Hypothesis holds that people with ADHD have a genetic predisposition to excel beyond the average neurotypical at various endeavors *when in a nurturing environment.*

I've written more about the theory in the entry *Having Reserves of Deep Potential* (in Part II), but suffice it to say there's some science behind the value I find in having someone nearby or with me when I'm working on certain things.

It's a branch of the same wisdom tree that has kids doing their homework together. Right? Or, having a personal trainer or walking, or working out, with a friend.

This is referred to as **body doubling.**

Having someone nearby who knows what you're doing (even if they're just sitting there reading a book) is like a psychological placeholder or ballast: Their presence holds you in place. Having someone there in the know about what you're doing helps you stay focused on your task and lessens the impulsive desire to fly off to something new.

Body doubling also helps overcome problems that would otherwise turn you off from making a start on something.

Like right now, I'm being psychologically crushed from having so many clothes in my closet that I never wear. But I cannot make myself work on it!

I'm going to need a friend to come sit with me and help me break through my resistance to purging the closet from too many items. I know there are many strategies for doing this (creating a giveaway bag; a throw-away bag: a stash-somewhere-for-a-year bag for items I can't bear to part with and will revisit in a year), but I can't face doing it alone. I need somebody here with me—even if they just sit around while I narrate what I'm doing.

Somehow, it's just so useful to have a mate nearby!

I love this service called Focus Mate (see *Resources*) where you can pair up with another person online for 50-minute work sessions. You don't talk beyond stating in the beginning what you'll be working on and saying goodbye at the end of the session. It's free for up to three sessions a week and charges a nominal fee for unlimited access.

Or if you know someone personally who wants to do this kind of body doubling, you can set up your own sessions on Zoom, Skype, or FaceTime.

Bookending

Bookending is a simple but powerful tool. It operates along the same principles as body doubling.

You call a trusted person before and after you do something that you're having a hard time getting done.

It's simple, but maybe not so easy. I often have a hard time picking up the phone. But maybe you don't!

This presupposes that you have a friend, coach, ADHD buddy, or other trusted pal who understands your challenges and supports you.

So that's it, that's all you do. You call them up and say, "Hey, quick call. I'm going to clean the kids' room for an hour. I'll call you back after I've done it. Thanks so much!"

Use a Therapist as an ADHD Coach

This is a simple suggestion: Use a therapist as an ADHD coach.

I used to think I had to use my time with a talking therapist to dig deep into my emotional health and troubling issues.

And, I've done quite a bit of that, and it's been extremely helpful for me (and I can imagine that the need may arise again in my life and I won't hesitate to go back to it).

But I realized, at one point, during a period when I wasn't seeing a therapist, that I could work with one strictly as an ADHD coach. So, I asked this woman I'd seen previously—who knew a lot about ADHD—and she was happy to do it. And, it was great. She helped me identify priorities; roughly schedule my work week; deconstruct projects into their action steps; stay accountable for what I had committed to doing; get back on track when I'd gone off, and more.

And, because I'm lucky enough to have good health insurance, each session only cost me a co-pay. Good deal.

Why not give it try?

Find Your Tribe

"I feel like I finally found my tribe! I have always been somewhat of an extrovert, and most definitely a people pleaser thanks to ADHD and childhood traumas, **but human connection is something I thrive on** *and so now I understand why I am drawn to certain types of people, why we connect so easily, and also why I sometimes forget about other people!"*

—Anastasia, wife and working mom

I love the book *Tribe: On Homecoming and Belonging*, by Sebastian Junger. **It's about the idea that much of what's so difficult for combat veterans transitioning back home is the loss of the daily community of platoon life.**

Junger, an experienced war correspondent, has seen the kind of horror that I don't even want to imagine. But he's also observed that even in the hell of war, the communal experience of living closely together (as soldiers do) creates a strong, comforting sense of belonging that fulfills the soldiers and makes everything better.

It's beyond ironic that something so deeply good can come from something so impossibly brutal. Yet it's true.

You can see the same sense of unity in communities after a natural disaster: the uplifting spirit that arises when people join together to help each other.

But there doesn't need to be a disaster to have your spirits lift from connecting closely in community with others like you. You don't have to live together in a barracks, either. You just have to connect with others, especially those who are in the same boat as you are, whatever that boat is. (Or, perhaps different boats, but the same river.)

The magic is in the coming together.

People are neurobiologically hardwired to connect with others and live with a sense of belonging.

Connecting is what we're doing here through the windows of this book.

I loved Junger's book because he validates this most potent of healing experiences.

I wish that there were as many mental health clubs out there as there are workout clubs.

When I hear about the isolation and depression of veterans transitioning back to American life, I die wishing that community groups were as widespread as coffee shops. I wish they were a fixture in our society—accepted as cool, not fringe, or weak, or hard to find. I wish they existed all over the place for all the depressed kids who fantasize about going on shooting sprees, and for the ones who have. I wish they existed without any stigma for suicidal kids and adults, and for all the drug and alcohol users. I wish they were all over the place like health clubs are. And free—or as cheap as Planet Fitness.

Somehow, we've got to find ways to create these places.

Awareness is the first step, right?

Ask for a Moment to Shift Gears

According to the writer M. Scott Peck, the ultimate act of love is giving another person your full attention.

And really, I try to do that when my husband starts going on and on about how some soccer player in another country's brother's wife's father started some organization or another. (My husband is a sportswriter.)

I really want to listen to him because it's a loving thing to do! And also because he listens to me talk my head off about my feelings on all kinds of things; my excitement about ADHD stuff; my spiritual experiences and quests; my beliefs about the nature of God and how, in an infinite universe, *anything at all is possible*, and all that.

Oh, but God, sometimes I just can't bear to listen to him without getting really irritated. So instead of pretending to listen and running the risk of turning nasty on him, I'll tell him that I'm sorry, but I just can't listen *now*—and can he tell me later? And when I'm really on my game, I'll say "Hey, I really want to hear this, but I can't right this minute."

On the other hand, if he starts talking about this stuff and I think that I can, in fact, unscrew my mind from what I'm doing and give him my attention, I'll ask him if he'll give me a minute.

And I take that minute (which might really be three or four minutes) and disengage from what I'm doing (online window shopping, LOL).

Then I might take that minute and go to the bathroom for a moment's privacy with myself and my little head.

In there, I might splash some water on my face and say to myself, "Ok! let's go listen to what this guy has to say. Someday, Joni, you're going to remember times like these as the good ol' days and wish you could be back here listening to him! Go do it!"

Which gets me appreciating the present moment and puts me in a state of receptivity to what he has to say. I'm unlikely to remember the details of this information-packed story that interests him so, but I follow it in the moment. Sometimes, it's more like I'm focused on his excitement and enthusiasm, rather than the actual facts of the story, but that's okay, I think. At least I will have been in there, in the moment, with him.

Which is all we ever have, right?

Take Notes

I take a lot of notes in a lot of situations, and I highly recommend it.

I still like longhand better than typing for quick stuff (even though I type really fast).

I keep my notebook with me and scribble key points when I'm on the phone with almost anybody.

I sometimes jot something down if something hits me in the night—sometimes even in the dark in big letters. So I always have my notebook and pencil on my bedside table.

I take notes when I'm on the phone with anybody about some household repair or inquiry; with a doctor's office; when making an appointment with anybody about anything. I ask questions and I get answers. I write all that stuff down.

Pretend you're a journalist and you need to get the story right.

Help With Interrupting

A number of triggers cause me to speak impulsively—that is, say something without thinking it through. Feeling excited or uplifted is a definite trigger: I'll feel buoyed by a conversation or experience and well up with a desire to share my excitement and rave about the matter at hand. Often, I find myself yelling (talking really loudly). Hopefully, you don't. But I do! I'm always apologizing about it and trying to lower my voice and calm my delivery down. I realized that I was doing it the other day and apologized to my friend. And her response was so fantastic: She said, "No! I love your enthusiasm!"

Still, not everybody reads my interruptions and loud voice as enthusiasm, and even if they are aware that I'm not angry or scolding, interruptions can really gum up the works—especially on the phone. **(It's hard on the phone because I'll interrupt and then the other person stops talking and I stop talking, and neither of us knows who should speak next, and that creates an awkward silence and messes up a flowing conversation.)**

So, because I want **to keep my interruptions to a minimum, I do a few things before and during a call or a meeting, party, or date.**

For one thing, I try to take a few minutes before the appointed event and remember my tendency to get very excited and that my intention is to modulate the expression of my excitement.

I create this intention either by thinking it through, saying it out loud or writing it down. I'll say, think, or write, "Joni, remember to stay as calm as you can and listen to the other person. Remember that you'll have your chance to say what you want. It'll be nice to talk to this person, and rest assured that you'll get your chance to say what you mean and feel."

I also sometimes wear an elastic band to play with and snap to remember.

When I do this, I'm careful not to put myself down for being highly excitable (being excited is a wonderful quality that lifts others up). Still, I seek to modulate the expression of my excitement so others will be able to read it as excitement and enthusiasm—instead of misreading it and thinking I'm angry or trying to shut them up.

If it's a phone call, or a business-type meeting, I make sure I have my notebook with me. This really helps because instead of interrupting when I have a comment I feel I just have to interject right then, I jot it down so I know I can bring it up later. This relieves the anxiety that sometimes causes me to interrupt.

In general, as a form of mental hygiene, I try to stay aware of specific times that my impulsivity has messed me up. I go over one or two such memories in my mind and nod my head yes.

Take the Best, Leave the Rest

I have to laugh when some ADHD specialist says, "Here, use this online calendar and sync it with your phone. Set alarms, etc." As if you could!

(I actually happen to be a techie, so I do this stuff and actually totally love it and depend on it.)

But so many people hate tech stuff, are confused by it, etc., so for them, it's not a good or useful suggestion. It's just annoying.

What works for one person can be useless (i.e., totally annoying) for another.

So take the best (tools/suggestions) and leave the rest, and try not to worry about the ones you can't use.

Use tools and strategies that "spark joy" in you. LOL!

Really, though, we're tackling challenges and uncovering assets, moment by moment. You might want to use one strategy every day for a week. Or for a month. If you used one strategy per month, you'd have 12 pretty solid tools at the end of a year.

And within each month, remember, there are about 30 days. Try to take them one by one: One day at a time.

One Last Thing

It's early August, 2023 and I'm almost done with the book you hold in your hands. I've been writing it for four years: all day some days, unable to even approach it on others.

I'm finding it very hard to let go and not keep adding things or trying to communicate what I mean more clearly!

I wrote my first short book as an experiment to see how to publish on Kindle. And it's been such a success (to me). I've reached thousands of women; heard such loving things from so many of you; and gotten hundreds of amazing online reviews which really helps the book sell so well.

As a journalist and writer, I'd always thought that the only legit way to have something published was by a reputable publication or publishing house. But the technological invention of **print on-demand publishing**—the ability for publishers to produce a single book when it's ordered—has changed all that.

Now, even agents from the big publishing houses recognize the power and reach of us "indie" authors!

Thank you for all for your support—all you women with ADHD. There are so many of us—so many mental health experts and laywomen communicating encouraging, uplifting, and helpful information online and in books.

I have no idea if this book will have the magic my first one has! I'm guessing that's unlikely since part of the allure of the other book is how short it is. We'll see. I've done my best and now it's time to leave the rest to the Universe. (Right?)

Looking back on these four years, which included the pandemic, I cannot believe that I had this much to say!

I'd be so happy to hear from any of you. I'm at joan.wilder@gmail.com.

Love,

JW

Resources

BOOKS

***A Radical Guide for Women with ADHD: Embrace Neurodiversity, Live Boldly, and Break Through Barriers*, Sari Solden, MS and Michelle Frank, PsyD**

Sari is a therapist and well-known expert on women with ADHD and seems to be a very warm woman and ADHDer herself. This, her newest book, written with Michelle Frank, is radical in the sense that it doesn't advise women to fix themselves, *but instead to learn to be themselves!* The book is especially helpful for women with inattentive ADHD, although its message of self acceptance and love is extremely helpful for all women with ADHD.

***ADHD 2.0: New Science and Essential Strategies for Thriving with Distraction—from Childhood through Adulthood*, by Edward M. Hallowell, M.D., and John J. Ratey, M.D.**

This is the latest book from this duo of doctors and ADHD experts who broke ground almost 40 years ago with the ADHD classic, *Driven to Distraction*. It is wonderfully short and extremely hopeful. It draws on Hallowell's years as a psychiatrist working with ADHDers at his Hallowell Centers, and Ratey's expertise in neuropsychiatry. Both are—or were—members of the Harvard Medical School and have vast experience studying and working with the ADHD brain. The book reflects the pair's compassionate and spirited view of ADHD, without denying its challenges.

Organizing Solutions for People With ADHD: Tips and Tools to Help You Take Charge of Your Life and Get Organized, (second edition), **by Susan C. Pinsky**

This woman is a professional organizer who has a genuine grasp of ADHD! Her approach to organizing for ADHDers developed from observing what her ADHD daughter needed to stay organized. It's a terrific book.

Living Daily With Adult ADD or ADHD: 365 Tips of the Day, **by Douglas A. Puryear, MD**

This is a very simple, helpful book with 365 short entries. Its contents are largely about strategies that Puryear has discovered to help him work through the daily difficulties he encounters—like driving off with the gas hose still attached to his car.

Help for Women with ADHD: My Simple Strategies for Conquering Chaos, **by Joan Wilder**

Hey, I had to put my first book in this list! It is only 60 short pages. (And, it has more than 1,000 wonderful reviews!)

Managing ADHD Workbook for Women: Exercises and Strategies to Improve Focus, Motivation, and Confidence, **by Christy Duan, MD, Kathleen Fentress Tripp, PMHNP-BC, Beata Lewis, MD**

This welcoming workbook, written by a trio of female mental health clinicians, offers women a comfortingly organized approach to ADHD's many parts through the friendly lens of its authors' experience. Each chapter has fill-in-the-blank sections aimed at helping readers apply its suggestions to their unique situations.

The Language of Letting Go: Daily Meditations for Codependents, **by Melody Beattie**

This 30-year best seller is filled with daily reflections about learning to care for ourselves and letting go of people-pleasing behaviors. Although it was written largely for the families of alcoholics and addicts, its wisdom transcends those identities. Growing up as an ADHDer in an environment that doesn't recognize, acknowledge, nurture, or accommodate an ADHDer's different nervous systems can leave us with some of the same problems and ingrained behaviors as people growing up, or living with, alcoholics/addicts.

Radical Acceptance: Embracing Your Life With The Heart of A Buddha, **Tara Brach, Random House LLC, 2004**

A beautiful book from Tara about awakening into the present from the trance of unworthiness most humans—whether or not they have ADHD—experience.

The Power of Your Unconscious Mind, Unlock the Secrets Within, **Joseph Murphy, Ph.D**

This is a much loved '60s-esque classic on how changing what you think can change your life. Murphy inspires readers to recognize that they have a source of intelligence within themselves that transcends the intellect and is more powerful. If you're at all open to affirmations, positive self-talk, the law of attraction, or other metaphysical teachings, definitely check out this book!

***Writing Down the Bones: Freeing the Writer Within*, Natalie Goldberg**

This book from 1986 introduced me to the idea of writing practice, i.e., putting pen to paper—for a set number of minutes or until you fill a set number of pages—and writing anything that comes to mind without judgement or censor. Later, Julia Cameron, who wrote the popular *Artist's Way*, reimagined Goldberg's writing practice in her recommendation that people write "morning pages:" three pages of free-flowing thoughts. I highly recommend this practice, aka, journaling, as a way to lessen many ADHDish traits, including overwhelm, lack of motivation, impulsivity, indecision, and more, whether you're a writer or not.

***Mini Habits: Smaller Habits, Bigger Results*, Stephen Guise**

After ten years of being unable to motivate himself to exercise no matter what he tried, Guise, one day in total frustration, asked himself if he could do one f*cking push-up. And he could, and he did. This evolved into his mini habit approach to getting motivated. The idea is to force yourself to do one tiny positive behavior every day that's so small and effortless that you can actually do it: Like his one push-up. And from that tiny effort, you get a tiny bit of fulfillment and forward motion, which is enough to power another push-up, and so on. A very encouraging book for ADHDers.

WEBSITES, MAGAZINES, ARTICLES, PODCASTS, SERVICES, AND OTHER RESOURCES

Attention Deficit Disorder Association (ADDA)
https://add.org

> This is a wonderful, 30-year-old non-profit dedicated to helping adults with ADHD. It's a storehouse for all kinds of information and services for people with ADHD, including courses, webinars, a couple dozen different ADHD virtual support groups, professional services, and more. A lot of the info is free at ADDA, or you can become a member (and unlock all of its content) for $7.60/month, or $79.97/year. You can also volunteer to work at ADDA (which could be a terrific way of connecting with others).

ADDitude Magazine
https://www.additudemag.com

> ADDitude Magazine delivers new articles every month on scientific and real-life topics pertaining to ADHD challenges.

ADHD Women's Palooza
https://adhdpalooza.com

> A fantastic annual online event that features dozens of interviews with ADHD experts. The talks are free when they are live, and can be accessed for money, even after the event is over. A huge resource for women with ADHD. Hosted by the effervescent ADHDer and gardener! Linda Roggli, PCC. Even if you've missed one year's Palooza, you can still access all the interviews and talks by buying them.

Inattentive ADHD Coalition

https://www.iadhd.org

> This nonprofit organization is focused on spreading information about the inattentive subtype of ADHD. Its mission is to ensure that all children and adults with inattentive ADHD be accurately diagnosed. The site is a great resource for ADHDers, especially if you're just learning about this subtype.

Psychology Today

https://www.psychologytoday.com/us

> The website for this magazine has an enormous directory of (talking) therapists. It's searchable by state. To have a look around, go to and click on *"Find a Therapist."*

Children and Adults with Attention Deficit Disorder (CHADD)

https://chadd.org

> This organization is a storehouse of information on ADHD for adults (as well as children). Look through the drop-down menus on the homepage for information on all aspects of ADHD as well as a comprehensive list of resources.

The ADHD Manual.com

https://theadhdmanual.com

> Although I find this site a bit confusing to navigate, it's filled with insightful thoughts about ADHD. It's the creation of Abby Chau, LMFT, ADHD-CCSP, a family therapist in Seattle who has ADHD. Click on *Tips and Tricks* to access more than 50 helpful podcasts Abby's made as she seeks to create

a life manual for ADHDers to replace our culture's neurotypical, one-size-fits-all "manual."

Tarabrach.com
https://www.tarabrach.com

Tara's site has a long listing of lovely, guided meditation talks, for free. She is the founder of Insight Meditation outside of Washington, D.C., and is also a therapist. (You can also put this site on your smart phone.)

Attention Deficit Disorder, The Official Open Facebook Group
https://www.facebook.com/groups/AttentionDeficitDisorderTheOfficialOpenGroup

This is a very helpful, active Facebook group where people share all kinds of things about ADHD.

Coming into Focus
https://www.harpersbazaar.com/culture/features/a41083545/adhd-in-adult-women/

An empowering article by Carla Ciccione in the Sept. 5, 2022 issue of *Harper's Bazaar* on the recent "epidemic" of women with ADHD.

Dr. Hallowell's Wonderful World of Different
https://drhallowell.com/listen/podcast/

This is a weekly podcast for thriving in our wired world with *NY Times* best-selling author, world-renowned ADHD psychiatrist, advocate, speaker, and ADHDer himself, Dr. Ned Hallowell, founder of The Hallowell Centers, located across the U.S., including ones in New York City, the Boston area,

California's Bay Area, and Seattle. And, with the advent of telehealth, you can connect with the centers from anywhere in the world.

FocusMate.com

https://www.focusmate.com

This service allows you to pair up with another person online for 50-minute work sessions. You don't talk, beyond stating in the beginning what you'll be working on and saying good bye at the end of the session. It's free for up to three sessions a week, and about $5 per month for unlimited sessions. There's a great, 30-second video that explains how it works on its very friendly website.

Linda Roggli, PCC, ADDiva Network

https://addiva.net

Roggli is the cofounder of the wonderful, annual online ADHD Women's Palooza, and a coach. Her site is fun.

Female ADHD Test

https://www.additudemag.com/self-test-adhd-symptoms-women-girls/

This is a simple self test for ADHD. It does not replace a clinical diagnosis but might be a first step for you. It may also help you list the experiences and ways of being you'll want to remember to tell a clinician when getting diagnosed, or a coach, when explaining the areas where you could use some support.

@ADHDLove2020

https://www.instagram.com/adhdlove2020/

> Yakini, the women behind this *Instagram* account, posts lots of very helpful, informative videos and interviews on a range of helpful ADHD issues. By checking who Yakini follows, you can find a whole tribe of ADHD women out there.

@xAdultingWithADHDx

https://www.instagram.com/xadultingwithadhdx/

> ADHD coach, Gloria Joy Sherrod, LCPC, is behind this very informative Instagram account. All her Instagram posts are reels and Sherrod is very articulate and engaging.

An Informal Index

A kid in a toy store, *19*
ADDCA Accredited ADHD & Life Coach Training Program, *131*
Addiction/alcoholism
    cannabis and me, *301*
    Higher than average incidence in ADHDers, *302*
ADHD
    accommodations, list of possible ones for ADHDers, *107*
    assets of, *73*
    subtypes of, *70*
ADHD 2.0, by Edward M. Hallowell, M.D., and John J. Ratey, M.D., *52*
Amygdala, *52*
Anecdotes from women with ADHD—in their words
    Alaina, *111*
    Anastasia, *143, 146, 161, 336*
    Bethenie, *34*
    Erika, *111*
    Gabi, *80, 108, 200, 233*
    Jessica, *77, 86, 99, 136*
    Joanne, *129*
    Julie, *30, 40, 104, 126, 203, 225*
    Mandy, *26, 303*
    Sara, *115, 156*
    Sarah, *96, 176*
    Selina Danielle, *40, 153, 262, 293*
    Yakini, *94, 194, 331*
Attention, one way to give it to another, *339*
Authentic self
    some ways it gets buried, *231*
    some ways to excavate it, *234*
Awareness
    how an ADHDer's is wide open, *80*
Balancing exercises
    as a possible help for ADHD, *52*
Beattie, Melody
    for help standing up for your feelings, *152*
Big picture thinking

An ADHD woman's
wholistic approach to a
problem, *35*
how it contributes to
invention, *88*
how we tend to jump right
into the middle of an
issue, *79*
Big rocks story, *208*
BLM
as example of need for
diversity, *105*
Brach, Tara, on humankind's
"trance of unworthiness",
108
Brain chemicals
role in ADHD, *24*
Brains, recognition that some
are good at some things,
others at other things, *228*
Brown, Brené, 167
CADDAC, Center for ADHD
Awareness, Canada, *132*
Cannabis
high incidence of use in
ADHDers, *301*
Cerebellum
its possible involvement in
ADHD and use in
alleviating its hard
traits, *52*
Cloninger, Dr. C. Robert
on factors for happiness,
96
Coach

Many links and directions
for finding an ADHD
coach and what they do,
131
Cohen, Leonard, 93
Conceptual expansion
A highly-prized ADHD
trait among those who
study invention, *87*
Connecting with others
The magic of connecting
with others, especially
those in the same boat,
337
The value to our health,
137
Cultural norms
societally agreed upon, *35*
Curiosity
for what's going on behind
the scenes, *81*
the value of, *96*
Death bed
thinking about yours as a
way to identify
priorities, *149*
Deeper cognitive experiences
How ADHDers think long
and deep about
everything, *64*
Diagnosis, titles of various
professionals who can
make one, *112*
Diagnostic criteria used to
diagnose ADHD

contained in the
Diagnostic and
Statistical Manual of
Mental Disorders
(DSM-5), *70*
Disagreeing in a healthy way
without taking or giving
offense, *327*
Divergent thinking
an ADHDer's strength at,
78
The ability to spin off
many ideas from a
single starting point, *78*
Diversity in nature
as a sign of health in an
ecosystem, *9*
Dodson, M.D., William, *226*
Dominant culture
as comprising a set of
expected behaviors that
marginalize
neurodivergent ways of
being, *106*
Dopamine. See
Neurotransmitters, role of
in ADHD
on low levels of it being
implicated in causing
ADHD, *24*
Educating others about
ADHD
some examples of what
you might say, *147*

Education for Persistence and
Innovation Center (EPIC),
166
Einstein, Albert quote, *77*
Encouragement and
recognition, 75
on its value to women with
ADHD, *75*
Environments
importance of for women
with ADHD, *25*
taking a self inventory to
identify which
environments are
stimulating to you, *225*
Estrogen
Its monthly dance, *144*
Failure, how the road to
success is lined with it, *166*
Filters, on ADHDers lacking
them, *19*
Fish, don't judge one by its
ability to run, *34*
Flooding, *51*
Focus, wide open in
ADHDers, *19*
Frontal cortex, *52*
Guise, Stephen, *258*
Hallowell ADHD Centers,
112, 132
Hallowell, M.D., Edward M.
on coining the Orchid
Hypothesis-like term
"Recognition Sensitive
Euphoria", *75*

Heads
- on how we're the only ones inside ours so please be nice, *290*

Heart, a woman's, *16*

Helping others, the value of giving and receiving, *330*

Hyperarousal, *19*

Ideas person, an ADHDer is an, *77*

Imagination, using yours to re-envision an event, *267*

Intelligence, the need to expand society's recognition of it, *36*

International ADHD Coach Training Center, The, *132*

Katie, Byron, *242*

Lao Tzu quote, *289*

Lateral thinking. See Divergent thinking

Lazy, ADHDers misunderstood as, *24*

LGBTQ, as example of diversity, *105*

Lying
- As soul crushing response to society's denial of neurodiversities as health issues, *328*

Medication, how it's lifesaving for many women with AHDH, *115*

Menopause, *144*

Mental/emotional issues as widespread in our culture, *90*
- how sharing about ours can help another person with theirs, *90*

Mini-habits, some examples of, *259*

Murphy, Joseph, *264*

National Institute of Mental Health, *70*

Negative emotions erupting quickly, *51*

Neurodivergent, meaning of, *105*

Neurotransmitters, role of in ADHD, *24*, *55*, *130*, *144*, *287*

Neurotypical, meaning of, *23*

Norepinephrine, *130*, *287*, See Neurotransmitters, role of in ADHD

Nouwen, Henri J.M., *89*

O'Reilly, Diane, ADHD Coach, *133*

Opinions, the damaging effect of hiding yours, *327*

Orchid and the Dandelion, The, by W. Thomas Boyce, M.D., *76*

Orchid Hypothesis, *76*

Outside the box thinking, *21*, *78*

P. Diddy, *46*

Patterns, on how ADHDers see connected, *80*

Peck, M. Scott, *339*
Perimenopause, *144*
Personal disarmament, *310*
Phone someone, as a way to connect, *139, 334*
PMS, its effects on ADHD, *144*
Prayer, *168*
Priorities, on how they help define what you want to live for, *149*
Psychologist Locator, The, *113*
Psychology Today, *113*
Puryear M.D., Douglas, one way to initiate a new habit, *274*
Queen of Distraction by Terry Maitland, BA, M.S.W, *114*
Ratey, M.D., John J., on coining the Orchid Hypothesis-like term "Recognition Sensitive Euphoria", *75*
Rejection sensitive dysphoria, *58*
Remifemin, *145*
Resentment, *309*
Resistance, *332*
Resume writing, as example of chunking, *209*
Review your day and imagine an event having gone differently, *267*
Rumi, the poet known as, *291*

Self esteem, *10*
Self inventory as a way to identify what motivates you, *226*
Self regulation, difficulty with, *51*
Sensitive perceivers, *20, 94*
Sensitive Person, Highly, *63*
Serotonin, *144, 287*, See Neurotransmitters, role of in ADHD
Shame, *108, 161*
Smaller Habits, Bigger Results by Stephen Guise, *258*
Solden, MS, Sari, on her belief that an ADHDer's self worth is distinct from her brain-based differences, *162*
Spectrum disorder
    One way to explain ADHD to others, *148*
Spectrum disorder, ADHD comprises a large umbrella of traits, *20*
Starting and stopping, *29*
Starting, difficulty with, *21, 291*
Stimulation, lacking, *24*
Surrender what you can't control, *296*
The Science of Success, *76*
Third place, find yours as a way to connect, *137*

Tribe: On Homecoming and Belonging by Sebastian Junger, *336*
Unfiltered focus, both sides of, *10*
Vestibulocerebellar system (VCS), possible role in ADHD, *52*

Wasserstein, Dr. Jeannette, as resource on women's hormones and ADHD, *145*
What to say when looking for a professional to diagnose you, examples of, *114*
Wheeler, Sarah, *228*
ZenCare, *114*

About the Author

As a freelance journalist, Joan Wilder has written hundreds of pieces that run the gamut from the hardest of hard news stories—fires, kidnappings, politics—to the most narrative of non-fiction features: travel stories, essays, and profiles. Her work has appeared in many magazines and daily newspapers, including the Boston Globe (she wrote weekly for the paper for more than a decade), and the Patriot Ledger, where she was a regular contributor with a beat for many years. She wrote "The Dish," a food column for Boston.com and reviewed hundreds of Boston-area restaurants for the Local section of the Globe (until the pandemic put an end to that). She's ghostwritten books and authored many other types of pieces: grants, press releases, book proposals, corporate newsletters, website copy, reference book histories, and narrative biographies. She is the author of the tiny book *Help for Women with ADHD: My Simple Strategies for Conquering Chaos (scan the QR code below to be taken to that book's web page.)* Please visit her at HelpForWomenWithADHD.com or joan.wilder@gmail.com (she'd be thrilled to hear from you!).

Printed in Great Britain
by Amazon